Taking Medicine

Women and Indigenous Studies Series

The series publishes works establishing a new understanding of Indigenous women's perspectives and experiences, by researchers in a range of fields. By bringing women's issues to the forefront, this series invites and encourages innovative scholarship that offers new insights on Indigenous questions past, present, and future. Books in this series will appeal to readers seeking stimulating explorations and in-depth analysis of the roles, relationships, and representations of Indigenous women in history, politics, culture, ways of knowing, health, and community well-being.

Other books in the series:

Being Again of One Mind: Oneida Women and the Struggle for Decolonization, by Lina Sunseri
Indigenous Women and Feminism: Politics, Activism, Culture, edited by Cheryl Suzack, Shari M. Huhndorf, Jeanne Perreault, and Jean Barman

Taking Medicine

Women's Healing Work and Colonial Contact in Southern Alberta, 1880-1930

KRISTIN BURNETT

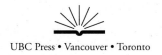

UBC Press • Vancouver • Toronto

© UBC Press 2010

All rights reserved. No part of this publication may be reproduced, stored in a retrieval system, or transmitted, in any form or by any means, without prior written permission of the publisher, or, in Canada, in the case of photocopying or other reprographic copying, a licence from Access Copyright (Canadian Copyright Licensing Agency), www.accesscopyright.ca.

20 19 18 17 16 15 14 13 12 11 10   5 4 3 2 1

Printed in Canada on FSC-certified ancient-forest-free paper
(100% post-consumer recycled) that is processed chlorine- and acid-free.

Library and Archives Canada Cataloguing in Publication

Burnett, Kristin, 1974-
  Taking medicine : women's healing work and colonial contact in Southern Alberta, 1880-1930 / Kristin Burnett.

(Women and indigenous studies series)
Includes bibliographical references and index.
ISBN 978-0-7748-1828-5 (bound); ISBN 978-0-7748-1829-2 (pbk.)

  1. Native women – Medical care – Alberta – History. 2. Women's health services – Alberta – History. 3. Native women – Health and hygiene – Alberta – History. 4. Women – Health and hygiene – Alberta – History. 5. Native peoples – Medicine – Alberta – History. 6. Native peoples – Medical care – Alberta – History. 7. Medical care – Alberta – History. I. Title.

RA450.A4B87 2010   362.1082'097123   C2010-902164-9

e-book ISBNs: 978-0-7748-1830-8 (pdf); 978-0-7748-5957-8 (epub)

Canada

UBC Press gratefully acknowledges the financial support for our publishing program of the Government of Canada (through the Canada Book Fund), the Canada Council for the Arts, and the British Columbia Arts Council.

This book has been published with the help of a grant from the Canadian Federation for the Humanities and Social Sciences, through the Aid to Scholarly Publications Program, using funds provided by the Social Sciences and Humanities Research Council of Canada.

A reasonable attempt has been made to secure permission to reproduce all material used. If there are errors or omissions they are wholly unintentional and the publisher would be grateful to learn of them.

UBC Press
The University of British Columbia
2029 West Mall
Vancouver, BC V6T 1Z2
www.ubcpress.ca

Contents

List of Illustrations / vii

Acknowledgments / ix

Introduction / 3

1 Niitsitapi: The Northwestern Plains / 17

2 Setting the Stage: Engendering the Therapeutic Culture of the Siksika, Kainai, Piikani, Tsuu T'ina, and Nakoda / 35

3 Giving Birth: Women's Health Work and Western Settlement, 1850-1900 / 47

4 Converging Therapeutic Systems: Encounters between Aboriginal and Non-Aboriginal Women, 1870s-90s / 67

5 Laying the Foundation: The Work of Nurses, Nursing Sisters, and Female Attendants on Reserves, 1890-1915 / 89

6 Taking over the System: Graduate Nurses, Nursing Sisters, Female Attendants, and Indian Health Services, 1915-30 / 121

7 The Snake and the Butterfly: Midwifery and Birth Control, 1900s-30s / 153

Conclusion / 169

Notes / 177

Bibliography / 213

Index / 229

Illustrations

2 / Map of southern Alberta and Treaty 7 communities

54 / Mrs. Adam Callihous, Hazelmere, 1955

62 / Mrs. John Bearspaw, Kew, 1916

72 / Grey Nuns, Blood Hospital, 1920s

77 / Mrs. Catherine Stocken, Blackfoot Reserve, 1890s

92 / Blood Hospital and pavilions, Standoff

93 / Blackfoot Hospital, late 1890s

99 / Nurses, Blackfoot Hospital, late 1890s

103 / Grey Nun, Blood Hospital

107 / Grey Nuns, Blood Hospital, 1930

115 / Nurse and pupils, St. Paul's Residential School, 1927

130 / Blood Hospital, Cardston, 1929

131 / DIA hospital, Morley, 1935

140 / Grey Nuns and DIA medical officer, Blood Hospital, 1930s

142 / Chapel, Blood Hospital, 1930s

150 / Baby show, Blackfoot Reserve, 1926

Acknowledgments

Many people contributed to the completion of this project and, without their support, this book would not have come to fruition. First and foremost, I have had the privilege of working with two exceptional feminist scholars: Kathryn McPherson and Sarah Carter. Kate was my doctoral supervisor and remains a valued friend and mentor. I am lucky to have met her. Sarah Carter supervised me during my master's degree at the University of Calgary and briefly as a postdoctoral fellow at the University of Alberta. She has consistently offered me good advice and support.

I would like to thank the following, in no particular order, for reading previous drafts of the work: William Wicken, Hugh Shewell, Megan Davies, Stephen Brookes, Christopher Armstrong, and Robin Jarvis Brownlie. All offered useful criticism and gave me a great deal to think about.

York University provided me with a stimulating and challenging intellectual community in which to develop. I want to thank Bettina Bradbury, Gina Feldberg, Craig Heron, Marcel Martel, Carolyn Podruchny, Anne Rubenstein, Myra Rutherdale, Marlene Shore, and William Westfall for their mentorship. I was also privileged to be part of an exciting graduate student community. In Toronto I met Daphne Bonar, Sarah Glassford, Christine Grandy, Ian Hesketh, Cynthia Loch-Drake, Sheila McManus, James Muir, Michele Stairs, Peter Stevens, Eric Strikwerda, and Karen Travers. I value their continuing friendship and intellectual support.

The staff at the Glenbow Archives, the Provincial Archives of Alberta, Library and Archives Canada, and the Saskatchewan Archives Board were very helpful and always answered my many questions with patience. In particular I would like to thank the Sisters of Charity. When I travelled to Montreal to examine the corporate records of the Grey Nuns at their motherhouse, the sisters welcomed me into their community and were very generous with their time and memories.

The editorial staff at UBC Press have been extremely helpful and patient, especially Darcy Cullen who helped me through every stage of the process. Without her guidance, this book would not have been possible. I want to thank Matthew Kudelka for his invaluable editorial expertise, and I want to express my sincere appreciation for the time, effort, and patience the anonymous readers put into examining my manuscript. They offered constructive and necessary criticism that helped me to improve the quality and the contribution of my work immeasurably. Special thanks are due to Jayne Elliot, who generously read the final manuscript to ensure that my medical terminology was clear.

My research benefitted from funding provided by Associated Medical Services, the Social Sciences and Humanities Research Council, and the Aid to Scholarly Publications Program.

In Thunder Bay I have had the great fortune to find a new community: Gail Fikis, Anna Guttman, Douglas Hayes, Catherine Hudson, Geoffrey Hudson, Patricia Jasen, Jane Nicholas, Jennifer Roth, Helen Smith, Victor Smith, Ben Stride-Darnley, Trish Sale, Pamela Wakewich, and Angie Wong-Hayes. I appreciate the friendship of Monica Flegel and her love of all things "supernatural"; Judith Leggatt, who helped me to find the convergence between my recreational and scholarly pursuits; and Lori Chambers, a very good friend, who read and commented on my manuscript. In particular I want to express my gratitude to my colleague and friend Bruce Strang, who welcomed me to Lakehead University, fed me frequently, offered me support and encouragement, and made me feel like part of his family. Thank you.

There are those friends who deserve particular attention, not only for their shared love of history but also for their sharp wit and humour, which helps me to keep things in perspective: Todd Webb, who is one of the smartest and funniest people I know and whose love of all things Methodist continues to confuse and amuse me; Carrie Lavis, who is like family; Lisa Rumiel, who coined the term *nap of denial*, is always willing to hang out and not work, and continues to be a real friend; Geoffrey Read, one of my closest and dearest friends, who is extremely generous with his time and is always willing to read a chapter and offer constructive criticism; and Chris Dooley, one of my favourite people and a constant source of encouragement, who shares my belief in the importance of space and place and is always willing to talk – I value our conversations and friendship.

I want to thank my family for their support and patience through this long process. I want to thank my uncle, Jim Burnett, whose own experiences in graduate school made him a sympathetic listener. I extend my sincere gratitude to the women in my family who have always given me encouragement and served as wonderful role models: Barbara Boissè, Vivian Burnett, and Jean Thivierge. To my mother, Christine Burnett, whose courage in the face of her illness has been a source of inspiration and strength, and to my brother, Steven, whom I love dearly and wish nothing but happiness.

Finally, I dedicate this book to the two most important men in my life. The first is Dylan Burnett, who was always there for me and left my life just as I was finishing this project. You are sorely missed. The second is my son, Adrian Thomas Burnett, who entered my life just as I was finishing the project. I love him, and he means everything to me.

Taking Medicine

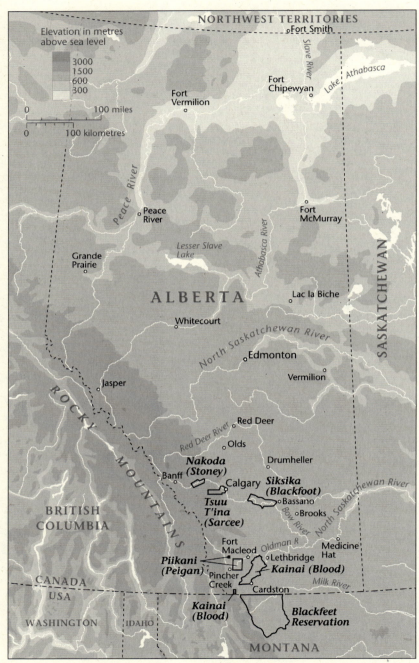

Map of southern Alberta and Treaty 7 communities | Cartographer: Eric Leinberger

Introduction

Aboriginal and Euro-Canadian women in western Canada were responsible for a diverse range of health care activities in Aboriginal and non-Aboriginal communities during the late nineteenth and early twentieth centuries. Aboriginal women who lived in what is now called the Prairie West (present-day Alberta, Saskatchewan, and Manitoba) possessed a great deal of expertise in midwifery and medicinal plants. This knowledge was essential to the well-being of both their own people and the newcomers who were settling in western Canada in increasing numbers. The Euro-Canadian women who came to live and work in the West after the 1870s, both as settlers and as missionaries, also brought with them varying degrees of expertise in Western healing and nursing practices. Both groups had formal therapeutic systems that were codified around precise treatments for specific illnesses, and this knowledge was transmitted from generation to generation in an orderly and circumscribed manner. Thus, when Aboriginal and non-Aboriginal women encountered each other, they, for a brief time, participated together in an informal system of healing and nursing care that drew on both traditions and centred on shared domestic concerns relating to childbirth and general childhood and family illnesses.[1] Over time, as the number of white settlers grew, the formal structures of Western medicine and nursing care increasingly dominated these more informal arrangements.

This study traces patterns of women's curative and caregiving work in a specific treaty area – that of Treaty 7 – across three generations, from the 1880s to the 1930s. In doing so it addresses important questions about gender, culture, and colonialism. First, an examination of Aboriginal women's curative and caregiving work in both Aboriginal and settler communities shows patterns of persistence, resistance, and change throughout these decades. Aboriginal culture was not a fragile entity, and though what constituted effective, necessary, and appropriate healing and medical care changed and was reimagined throughout this period, it was always understood within an existing cultural framework.[2] In other words, although the everyday practices of healing might have been modified, the underlying cultural values, meaning, and goals that characterized how Treaty 7 people and practitioners dealt with and understood health and well-being remained the same. Indeed, exposure to new diseases required Aboriginal peoples to develop new therapies, to use existing botanical medicines and treatments in different ways, and to incorporate elements of Western biomedicine that proved effective against particular illnesses. The adoption of certain elements of Western medicine by Aboriginal women did not signify cultural disintegration; rather, it was a pragmatic response to changing social, economic, and political conditions. Within this framework of survival and adaptation, Aboriginal women performed important health care functions in their communities – and to a lesser extent among non-Aboriginal people – well into the 1930s.

Second, Euro-Canadian women did much to establish Western-style medical systems on reserves and in the Prairie West more generally. The emergence of colonial health care regimes in Treaty 7 communities during the final decades of the nineteenth century coincided with the gradual transformation of nursing in Canada into a respectable profession carried out predominantly by trained middle-class white women.[3] Important developments in the professionalization of nursing through education and regulation occurred in the late nineteenth and early twentieth century. Health care undertaken by untrained or partially trained women with varying degrees of skill, experience, and respectability was gradually taken over by a cadre of educated women licensed by the Province of Alberta. On Treaty 7 reserves, this so-called professionalization process took place more gradually and was shaped by the broader assimilative goals of both the churches and the state.

Examining a specific treaty area brings the activities of non-Aboriginal female health workers into sharper focus. Euro-Canadian women, both as untrained attendants and as graduate nurses, did much to help establish the federally funded Indian Health Services (IHS) in 1928. The IHS was a key element in the colonization of Aboriginal peoples. After Treaty 7 was negotiated in 1877, the federal government and its employees solidified their control over Aboriginal peoples in southern Alberta, and Euro-Canadian women were caught up in this process, especially through their health care work, first as mission workers and later as government employees.

In some ways the medical facilities established on Treaty 7 reserves operated under the same patriarchal and hierarchical regimes that characterized hospitals and staffs in white communities. However, social and physical isolation combined with the absence of male medical professionals and the influence of the church ensured that female health workers on reserves, trained and untrained, carried out their work under different conditions than their urban counterparts. Reserve health workers sometimes made treatment decisions far beyond their level of training; at other times, Euro-Canadian nurses were required to navigate multiple and often conflicting levels of authority to achieve not only the best treatments for their patients but also workplace autonomy.

Third and finally, during the decades this book examines, the healing expertise of Aboriginal women served as a means of cultural exchange between Aboriginal people and Euro-Canadians, especially the women of both groups. The need for health care and nursing in the Prairie West helped develop a space where women came into contact with one another through shared domestic health concerns. These moments were not typically sustained but ended as soon as the crisis or illness passed. But sometimes these exchanges were repeated over long periods – for example, when a local Aboriginal woman came to be relied on by white settler communities for her healing powers or when two individuals came to rely on each other over many decades. However great the geographical and social distance between Aboriginal and non-Aboriginal women during this period, these women sought one another out in times of need and illness at locations that ranged from camps and farmhouses to dispensaries and hospitals. Colonialism and its internal (read "intimate" or "domestic") applications were still very much in effect in these locations, but to see this clearly we must, as historian Linda Gordon urges, turn our "attention to relations not always visible."[4]

In the early decades of white settlement in the West, the healing expertise of Aboriginal women produced brief moments of connection between Aboriginal and non-Aboriginal people. The expansion of white settlement and of Western health care eventually, and in fundamental ways, transformed relations between Aboriginal and Euro-Canadian people, especially women. Euro-Canadian women played significant roles in the founding of Western health care regimes on Treaty 7 reserves, both as front-line workers and as agents of social change. After 1900 the important therapeutic work performed by Aboriginal women became less and less visible. Indeed, the health of Aboriginal communities and the use of biomedicine became standards by which the progress of Aboriginal people was measured and contested. As front-line health care, social service, and educational workers, Euro-Canadian women mediated, administered, and adjudicated many of the experiences Aboriginal peoples had with the colonial state. Yet the healing and midwifery skills of southern Alberta's Aboriginal women continued to be viewed as important resources, despite the growth of Western medical services. Perhaps this was because of continued demand in impoverished communities. By focusing on the health work of women in the Treaty 7 area and among specific Aboriginal groups – the Blackfoot Nation, consisting of the Kainai (Blood), the Siksika (Blackfoot), and the Piikani (Peigan), as well as the Tsuu T'ina (Sarcee) and Nakoda (Stoney) – this book provides a more complicated picture of the state's impact on areas such as health and of the different ways women responded to and were affected by colonialism.

Western medical institutions and the health care work of Euro-Canadian women were at the heart of the colonial project in southern Alberta. As in so many other colonial locales, the Catholic and Protestant churches and their various missions built hospitals, school infirmaries, and dispensaries during the 1890s, the purpose of which was, as they saw it, to civilize Aboriginal peoples. These missions relied on Euro-Canadian women to operate the medical facilities and to provide domestic instruction to Aboriginal women. To fund these facilities and programs, the churches approached Ottawa, which found itself drawn reluctantly into financing a growing patchwork of medical institutions and services. After 1915 the Department of Indian Affairs (DIA) began to take direct control of mission facilities and programs. Euro-Canadian women remained the primary workers for both the churches and the state because they were an affordable and dedicated labour force; in addition, their gender allowed them entry into domestic sites believed to be in desperate need of improvement.

In western Canada, as elsewhere, the colonization of Aboriginal peoples and cultures resulted in close links between church and state. Missionaries were at the forefront of producing what Jean and John Comaroff refer to as a "state of colonialism."[5] The cultural interventions of missionaries – transforming people's perceptions, changing material habits, and reforming rituals – paved the way for later state interventions. Female missionaries in southern Alberta worked as trained and untrained health workers and ran instructional programs for Aboriginal women. After 1915 this work was increasingly taken over and managed by female government employees and public health nurses. The relationships that missionary women formed with Aboriginal women were different from those formed by female DIA employees. Missionaries spent years – indeed, often decades – living and working on reserves. Lay health workers did not. Female missionaries opened their homes to Aboriginal women and children. They regularly cared for them during times of illness and taught them to cook or knit in their own kitchens. In contrast, government employees were often stationed for only short periods, and there were fewer of them. In some ways, the intimacy that missionary women developed with Aboriginal women made their activities all the more insidious because the intentions of female Euro-Canadian mission workers were more opaque than those of their counterparts in the civil service.

Although the government was willing to fund this patchwork of mission-run health facilities and workers, these programs had little impact on the overall health and well-being of Aboriginal communities. The presence of Western health care facilities and female workers did not address real problems, which were rooted in poverty and colonialism. Historians Mary-Ellen Kelm and Maureen Lux – whose research focuses on British Columbia and the Prairie West, respectively – have explored the relationship between rates of morbidity and mortality and poor rations, insufficient clothing, and inadequate housing.[6] Both scholars describe the impact of economic and social dislocation that took place in Aboriginal communities during the late nineteenth century. Confined to reserves, cut off from hunting and gathering activities, and subjected to the harsh governance of federal authorities, Aboriginal people were less able to combat and rebound from ill health. Material deprivation led to a rise in diseases associated with poverty, malnutrition, and poor living conditions, such as tuberculosis.

This study builds on the work of Lux and Kelm by focusing specifically on the healing work of Aboriginal women, female medical missionaries, and white graduate lay nurses, in the early and informal network of healing and caregiving in western Canada and in the colonial medical regimes that developed after the 1890s. I seek to foreground women's therapeutic work not only as part of cultural persistence, resistance, and change in Aboriginal communities but also as an integral part of western settlement and the creation of colonial regimes.

Since the late 1980s, scholars have increasingly recognized women's place as both colonizers and colonized in the colonial project. They have identified gender as a central component in the operation of colonialism. It is now clear that understandings of femininity and masculinity were essential to the creation of sites of difference and meaning. The bodies of women and the works they performed in both public and private space were always at centre stage and did much to inform how opposing cultures viewed and reacted to one another. In the Treaty 7 area, racial differences were embodied first in domestic, medical, and healing practices and beliefs. Later, after the DIA health regime was created, those same differences were embodied in the strictures of Western medicine and in what the colonizers viewed as appropriate domestic and personal hygiene.[7] In this way, women's bodies and their domestic skills came to be the focus of state efforts to transform Aboriginal society. For female missionaries and DIA employees, "ideas of cleanliness, sanitation and middle-class white material culture were conflated as the indicators of Christian belief and 'civilized' behaviour."[8]

Examining the range of medical, healing, and nursing care interactions that took place between Aboriginal and Euro-Canadian people, especially women, also opens a path to consider a more complex network of social relations in the West. White settler societies did not suddenly appear fully formed. Rather, these societies developed in ways that reveal how gendered and racial categories are constantly reworked when encounters take place between different cultures and peoples. In western Canada, women's bodies might have served as boundary markers in an official and discursive capacity between Aboriginal and non-Aboriginal people. But at the same time, the experience of living in the West required that boundaries be transgressed in very personal and intimate ways, especially with regard to childbirth and family illnesses. As anthropologist and historian Ann Laura Stoler correctly points out, it was in the domestic intimacies of daily life that "colonial regimes of truth were imposed, worked around ... worked out," and often bound in "codes of silence."[9] The work that Aboriginal women did in the homes of white settlers remains largely unacknowledged in the narrative of settlement.

A broad range of interactions took place between the peoples of western Canada over a century of contact, as elsewhere in the colonial world. As colonizers, the arriving Europeans set out to establish a white settler society with white women as mothers of the race.[10] But given the remoteness of the Prairie West, how were white women supposed to give birth to a white society when they were far from traditional support networks, including midwifery care? To help answer this question, we should consider Stoler, who rejects the "fixity of racial categories" and instead explores how identities were set and then reconfigured in the colonial context. A Blackfoot woman could well find herself welcome in the home of a white rancher as a healer but prohibited from walking the streets of Medicine Hat or Lethbridge without a pass. Colonial categories were social concepts – that is, they were "provisional rather than placeholders and subject to review and revision," depending on the circumstances.[11] This was especially true in colonial settings, where gender complicated categories of race. As historian Anne McClintock aptly observes, because colonial women were "barred from the corridors of formal power, they experienced the privileges and social contradictions of imperialism very differently from colonial men."[12] The danger of giving birth in the harsh environment of the West required white women to seek help from the very people they were trying to dispossess. This paradox reveals, first, the contradictions of the colonial project and, second, that women's bodies were "often bound up in creating and perpetuating an often hidden complex, contradictory, and fraught history."[13]

Re-examining the spaces where women from different cultures met is extremely important because these encounters challenged Euro-Canadians' preconceived assumptions and stereotypes about Aboriginal women.[14] In her work on female missionaries in the North, historian Myra Rutherdale found that the very nature of the mission field – that is, the social isolation and the physically harsh environment – created ambiguity in the relationships between the missionaries and Aboriginal people.[15] This study reveals that a similar situation existed in western Canada: women who lived in isolated and remote regions looked for other women to assist them during childbirth, regardless of their cultural background or practices.

White women, as missionaries or settlers, did not compel Aboriginal women to adopt their own cultural preferences; instead, the West demanded a great deal of accommodation and collaboration between cultures. In her examination of Euro-Canadian women in the North, Barbara Kelcy contends that geographical isolation and a sparse white settler population limited the influence that white women had on Aboriginal peoples.[16] In the late 1800s, white settlement in southern Alberta and southwestern Saskatchewan was sparse, and white settlers were outnumbered by the local Aboriginal population until the 1890s. As a result, Euro-Canadian women were forced to accept the help of Aboriginal women. The Canadian west offers a wealth of examples that show how Aboriginal women assisted female colonists, sharing information with them regarding the environment and its resources.[17] These interactions reveal the inherent contradictions present in white settler communities. Boundaries between Aboriginal and non-Aboriginal people were fluid, and this mutability was especially evident in the encounters women had that involved health and healing.

This is not to suggest that these encounters were free of anxiety or that they ameliorated unequal power relations. Anxieties about race were often reactions to the complex relationships that had developed in western Canada – relationships that seemed to produce porous rather than fixed social categories. The diversity of mixed-race relationships in colonial locales, and their sheer number, provoked a great deal of unease regarding white men's claims to morality, manliness, and racial superiority.[18] In British Columbia, missionaries and civic leaders tried to temper interactions between Aboriginal and Euro-Canadian people through legislation and social censure. Likewise, in Calgary, municipal authorities tried to prevent Aboriginal women from traversing city streets, in the belief that they threatened social order and morality.[19] An examination of local newspapers revealed that similar concerns were never raised about Aboriginal women placing their hands on white women during childbirth or working as domestic servants in settlers' homes. Department of Indian Affairs annual reports applaud the domestic work of Aboriginal women in the homes of ranchers as they entirely overlook their midwifery work. Economic geographer Linda McDowell notes that "domestic space is the material representation of the social order"; consequently, because the "domestic help" of Aboriginal women took place in the home rather than in public space, the presence of Aboriginal women was not viewed as threatening or subversive. It instead reproduced Euro-Canadian visions of a white settler society and Aboriginal women's place within it.[20]

This book examines the healing work of the Siksika, Kainai, Piikani, Tsuu T'ina, and Nakoda women of southern Alberta from the 1880s to the 1930s. Focusing on a particular treaty area and its five reserves shows how the colonial experience was gendered, how it operated differently for different groups, and how even within the administrative limits delineated by the treaties, disparities continued to exist between reserves in terms of policy, personnel, and access to services. Although Treaty 7 remains the primary geographical focus of this work, there are times, particularly in the first and second chapters, when this study's geographical boundaries expand and contract. I adopted this practice for a number of reasons. First, the provinces of Alberta and Saskatchewan were created in 1905 and, thus, are relatively recent constructs. Second, before the treaties were negotiated and the reserves were settled, present-day boundaries meant little to the people of the Prairie West. Third, the fragmented and Eurocentric nature of the source materials required me to draw from a larger geographical area to discern a pattern. And fourth and finally, there are enough similarities relating to the progress and nature of settlement among different regions in prairie Canada over time that comparisons can be drawn.

There is no universal term for Aboriginal people in North America.[21] In Canada, the term *Aboriginal people* collectively refers to the original people of North America and their descendants "without regard to their separate origins and identities." I have chosen to use the term *Aboriginal people(s)* – which comprises Indian, Métis, and Inuit – because it is a more inclusive term (the Prairie West contained many different cultures and groups that do not fit under the rubric *First Nations*).[22] Moreover, because the documentary records (settlers' narratives, travellers' accounts, and so on) that describe the curative and caregiving aid offered by Aboriginal women do not identify whether individuals or groups belong to specific nations – the term *Aboriginal people* is appropriate. When sources (both written and oral) allow, I refer to specific nations and bands.

To understand the roles that Aboriginal and Euro-Canadian women played in this era of state building, colonization, and Aboriginal survival and resistance, this study draws from a wide range of primary sources. Each type demanded careful reading because of the ways in which gender and race combined to produce the record. This is especially true for primary materials pertaining to Aboriginal women. The Aboriginal peoples of the northwestern Plains, especially the Blackfoot, were among the most closely studied Aboriginal groups in twentieth-century North America. Much of the interest was propelled by the imagery of the buffalo hunter, whose masculine traits came to represent the classic Indian in the imagination of North American people.[23] Within this source base, Aboriginal women rarely appear. Anthropological accounts, memoirs, oral histories, local histories, and government and church records must therefore be read carefully for the glimpses of Aboriginal women's lives they contain. Except for certain oral history materials, these sources were produced almost entirely by Europeans, with marginal Aboriginal participation.

In contrast to their Aboriginal counterparts, white women had more opportunities to pen their own histories, be these first-person accounts or entries in institutional and organizational records. Still, government records are surprisingly silent on many aspects of white women's work and often foreground the roles of professional men such as doctors or government officials such as Indian agents. Because of the challenges posed by the primary resources, this study draws from a wide range of materials and seeks to use each type carefully by situating them in the context of the political and social world in which they were produced.

Interviews were not conducted for this study. In the current political and social climate of southern Alberta, many members of Treaty 7 are reluctant to talk because treaty litigation is ongoing. In addition, they are largely tired of the constant scrutiny of researchers, and few people are alive who are old enough to remember the period prior to 1940. I instead rely on oral history collections that have been completed by other researchers over the past thirty years. This oral history material is especially useful for allowing us to hear the voices of Aboriginal people in a historical record dominated by Europeans.

Published and unpublished sources serve as important complements to the oral history material. Over the past twenty years, a number of memoirs of individuals associated with Treaty 7 have been published, in part to address the lack of Aboriginal voices in the historical record and in part to document the memories of elders before their cultural knowledge is lost. These works, like the oral history materials, speak to contemporary political and economic struggles in Aboriginal communities, especially those issues dealing with land claims and treaty rights. There are also a substantial number of published and unpublished memoirs of settlers and retired government officials. These accounts reflect Euro-Canadian experiences within the broader story of the West's settlement. They are structured around a broader narrative of development, progress, the advance of civilization, and the marginalization of Aboriginal cultures. Yet they also contain candid reflections of daily life.

Anthropological texts and field notes pose a similar challenge. In the late nineteenth and early twentieth centuries, ethnographers and anthropologists – many of them amateur – spent a great deal of time living and working among the Aboriginal peoples they studied. These observers were in many ways participants in Aboriginal culture. They relied on interviews with Aboriginal people to secure information about cultural practices, and some of them, such as Clark Wissler, used Aboriginal men to perform fieldwork.

Franz Boas, often considered the father of American anthropology, initiated profound changes in North American anthropology.[24] As a professor at Columbia University, he accelerated a shift from anthropology as a part-time hobby to anthropology as a discipline practised by academically trained natural scientists concerned with the collection of hard data.[25] Of course, Boas was not alone in encouraging the professionalization of anthropology: academics in England, Germany, and even New Zealand were developing their own anthropological traditions. In Canada, the work of New Zealand–educated Diamond Jenness has been especially important. Jenness received a degree in anthropology in 1910 under the supervision of R.R. Marett. During his first five years in Canada (from 1913 to 1918), he collected and organized anthropological data for the southern party of the first Canadian Arctic Expedition, organized by Vilhjalmur Stefansson. Although Jenness is best known for his work among Inuit, during the summer of 1922 he spent two months doing field research among the Tsuu T'ina.[26]

Whether written by amateurs or professionals, published anthropological reports often include only limited discussions of women's work. Yet many anthropologists' unpublished field notes document a range of practices and activities that are not included in the published texts. Those anthropologists who performed fieldwork during the 1930s left behind unedited field notes, and discussions of childbirth and birth control figure quite prominently in them. The original copies of these notes are housed in a range of North American repositories, and the Glenbow Archives in Calgary has copies of them. The acquisition reflects Glenbow Archive's resolve, in co-operation with Treaty 7 communities, to locate and house these materials. Unfortunately, the field notes from Jenness' two-month stay among the Tsuu T'ina have not survived.

To outline the history of Western health care regimes in Aboriginal communities, this study utilizes the records of the DIA and of the churches and their affiliated missionary organizations. Department of Indian Affairs records tend to foreground the work of male medical professionals. The nursing care provided by female workers – which was often the bulk of day-to-day medical care – is not described directly and can only be inferred. Still, the sheer volume of correspondence and reports generated by the DIA reveals the shape that Western medical services took, the federal government's objectives, and what the DIA regarded as necessary and appropriate medical treatment for Aboriginal people.

The records of the churches and their affiliated missionaries are invaluable because they help make visible the work of female health care providers. In some ways the reports and letters of church and mission employees were more self-promotional than those produced by DIA employees because missionaries needed the financial support of congregations in eastern Canada. This meant that missionaries – especially female ones – had to show there was a real need for their work. Since Euro-Canadian women could not perform the rite of conversion, their importance in the mission field lay in the social services they provided – in particular, nursing care. The records of missionary organizations contain some of the few descriptions and letters produced by Euro-Canadian women on reserves. Descriptions of day-to-day nursing labour are embedded in the letters these women wrote to missionary societies.

Access to church records for this book presented a particular challenge. The Anglican Church is facing litigation because of its administration of residential schools and has been very cautious about opening its records to researchers. The records for the Anglican Church, Calgary Diocese, are stored in a number of places. A few decades ago, several churches within the Calgary Diocese donated their records to the Glenbow Archives. This record group contains almost five years of reports from the nurses stationed at the Tsuu T'ina Reserve – an unusual find. Subsequently, in 2002, before the remainder of the Calgary Diocese records were deposited at the University of Calgary, a careful culling of the materials was undertaken. As a result, parish records documenting births and deaths and materials pertaining to health conditions in residential schools are incomplete, making it impossible to chart precisely the health status of Aboriginal people who lived in Anglican parishes.

I faced similar restrictions researching Catholic parishes. The Sisters of Charity, who hold baptismal and death records for the southern Alberta region, refused to provide access to those records. The order did, however, grant access to the institutional records and correspondence produced by the sisters at the Blood Hospital, especially those materials written by the sister superior and the reverend general at Nicolet. In return for being allowed access to this source base, I promised I would not publish personal information about any of the sisters or use their real names.

At the end of the day, despite the broad and diverse record base I relied on, it is difficult to "know" Aboriginal women. Most of the records used for this study are ethnocentric and patriarchal in tone, and they really only tell part of Aboriginal women's stories. But I hope this is not simply another history of colonizing whites gazing at the Other. These types of interpretations imply that Aboriginal women did not have volition. I suggest that we can catch glimpses of the curative work performed by Aboriginal women – not the mindset or the intention, but the work. The curative and caregiving work of both Aboriginal and white women was vital to Aboriginal and newcomer communities in the late nineteenth and early twentieth centuries. But as white settlement expanded along with Euro-Canadian institutions, the work of Aboriginal women was displaced. Within the health care framework that developed in western Canada after the 1890s, Euro-Canadian women were important. They helped establish colonial medical regimes on Treaty 7 reserves. The healing work of Aboriginal women did not disappear, but it struggled to survive the challenges it faced under the weight of the colonial state.

Chapter 1 outlines the history of the Siksika, Kainai, Piikani, Tsuu T'ina, and Nakoda peoples. Chapter 2 examines the healing skills and knowledge that were the domain of Aboriginal women in the late nineteenth and early twentieth centuries. Chapter 3 extends the examination of Aboriginal women's healing work to the curative skills that Aboriginal women made available to newcomers – in particular, to the white women who participated in the founding of white settler colonies in western Canada. Chapter 4 looks at the growing presence of missions and missionaries in southern Alberta. In this period the mission house and the healing and nursing care provided by mission women became part of the therapeutic strategies followed by Aboriginal people. Chapter 5 shifts the focus to the evolving institutional structures of Western medicine in Aboriginal communities. Euro-Canadian women played a key role in these institutions because they were a cheap source of labour dedicated to working among Aboriginal people. The work of missionary nurses laid the foundations for the state-run apparatus that emerged in the years surrounding the First World War. Chapter 6 examines the federal government's gradual takeover of health services in southern Alberta and emphasizes the role of nurses in DIA hospitals, clinics, and public health programs. By the 1930s the shape that IHS would take for the next several decades was in place.

The final chapter comes full circle to look at the persistence of Aboriginal women's healing work, especially midwifery, in their communities in the twentieth century. Throughout the 1920s growing numbers of Aboriginal women made use of DIA institutions for confinement and childbirth, but they did not entirely abandon Aboriginal curative, caregiving, midwifery, and reproductive practices. Rather, the women of southern Alberta's Aboriginal communities drew from a range of Aboriginal and Western health care strategies as they struggled to sustain their families and culture.

I

Niitsitapi

The Northwestern Plains

This study is framed by the geographic, political, economic, and social boundaries created by Treaty 7 after 1877. But to understand the gender-specific nature of northwestern Plains peoples' healing practices and the interactions of those practices with European ones, it is necessary to understand the place of curative regimes in the broader region's history and economy.

THE FIRST PEOPLES

The five tribes that currently reside in the Treaty 7 area – Tsuu T'ina and Nakoda and the three tribes of the Blackfoot Nation (Siksika, Kainai, and Piikani) – contain further divisions. The Piikani are divided geographically into North and South Piikani, and the South Piikani live in Montana and are referred to as the Blackfeet. These current divisions reflect the drawing of national boundaries in the nineteenth century and the efforts of Aboriginal people to negotiate dramatic social, political, and economic changes.[1]

The Blackfoot language belongs to the Algonquian family. According to archaeologists, the Blackfoot were originally an Eastern Woodlands people.[2] They were probably the first group to arrive on the northwestern Plains, and there is physical evidence that they were present in southern Alberta as early as the 1550s.[3] By the late eighteenth and early nineteenth centuries, the Blackfoot Nation encompassed an enormous area, bounded on the west by the Rocky Mountains, on the north by the North Saskatchewan

River, and on the east by the present-day Alberta-Saskatchewan border. The nation extended as far south as the Missouri River.[4]

The Tsuu T'ina, an Athapaskan-speaking people, originated in the Canadian subarctic. An offshoot of the Tsattine (Beaver) of present-day northern Alberta (near Lesser Slave Lake), the Tsuu T'ina split from the Tsattine sometime between 1700 and 1750 as a result of the fur trade's westward expansion.[5] Incursions into the region north of the North Saskatchewan River by groups of Cree hunters armed with guns drove the Tsuu T'ina farther and farther south onto the parklands and foothills of present-day southern Alberta.[6] The animosity the Tsuu T'ina and the Blackfoot shared toward the Cree helped solidify an alliance between the two groups. When the Tsuu T'ina moved out onto the plains of southern Alberta, they adopted a lifestyle similar to that of the Blackfoot. They copied their social organization, military societies, and religious practices.[7] Yet they also held on to their language and their separate tribal identity.

The Nakoda (Assiniboine) were originally part of the Yaktonai Dakota (who in turn were part of the Sioux-Nakoda Nation). Internal conflict led to a split between the Assiniboine and the Yaktonai Dakota. The Assiniboine moved north into the territory around the Lake of the Woods and Lake Winnipeg, where they became allies of the Cree. The Assiniboine were highly active as go-betweens in the fur trade and, as that trade shifted farther west, the Assiniboine followed it, spreading west across the Plains into Saskatchewan and Alberta as well as south into Montana.[8] As certain kinds of fur-bearing animals became scarce, the Assiniboine modified their role within the fur trade. Instead of trapping and trading furs, they began supplying trading posts with dried meat and pemmican.

By the 1700s several small Nakoda bands had separated from the Assiniboine and migrated as far west as the Rocky Mountains. Some of these bands lived in the woodlands and foothills; others moved out onto the Plains and hunted buffalo.[9] During the 1860s and 1870s, the Nakoda divided into three bands: Bearspaw, Chiniki, and Goodstoney. The Bearspaw band hunted the southern portion of Nakoda territory, travelling south into Montana to hunt buffalo. To the north, the Chiniki band hunted the area around present-day Banff National Park. The Goodstoney band lived in the woodlands near the headwaters of the North Saskatchewan.[10] The Goodstoney and Chiniki bands continued to hunt buffalo, but elk, moose, and deer were their primary source of animal protein. Today, these three groups reflect contemporary band membership and residence among the Nakoda in southern Alberta.

Despite important historical, cultural, and linguistic differences among the peoples of the northwestern Plains, by the nineteenth century they shared a common economic structure that was heavily influenced by local environment. The northwestern Plains are largely flat, treeless, and arid and are subject to extreme and fluctuating temperatures.[11] The seasonal availability of plants and the migration of the buffalo determined Plains peoples' annual cycle of journeys. In the winter they gathered in small bands along wooded river bottoms near the foothills. In the spring they moved out onto the prairies.[12] Recent work by archaeologists Mary Malainey and Barbara Sheriff offers evidence that buffalo herds wintered on the open prairie, and so too did the people who hunted them.[13]

The buffalo were extremely important to the economy of the Blackfoot, Tsuu T'ina, and Nakoda. Buffalo were more than just a food source: they supplied the northwestern Plains peoples with shelter, fuel, clothing, bedding, containers, and tools.[14] Nevertheless, given the "unpredictable alternation of abundance and scarcity" that was characteristic of a reliance on buffalo, survival and prosperity in this region meant locating and drawing from a wide variety of animal and plant resources. Women's knowledge of the local environment was therefore vital.[15] Aboriginal women gathered and preserved a range of plants, roots, and berries throughout the year. These harvesting activities ensured that Plains people had a mixed diet. They also cushioned communities against times of scarcity.[16] Women's harvesting activities would remain an important part of the household economy in the West. Throughout the late nineteenth and early twentieth centuries, newcomer women who helped their husbands establish farms on the northwestern Plains found it necessary to rely on local plants and roots to feed their families.[17] And these women acquired their botanical knowledge from Aboriginal women.

Bands organized themselves in ways that ensured the community's survival. The band was the smallest political unit of the tribe and consisted of many unrelated nuclear families who formed groups on the basis of friendship and co-operation rather than kinship. The size of a band was flexible and could number anywhere from one hundred to three hundred. Generally, though, a band was small enough to find food for all its members but large enough to ensure safety from enemy attacks.[18] Bands split up and reconstituted themselves for a variety of economic, political, and social reasons. For example, the availability of food and other resources often determined band size. A successful bison drive required at least one hundred people.[19] During the nineteenth century, other factors, such as epidemics, also affected the number of bands, their membership, and their size.[20]

Religious and spiritual activities also influenced band movements and group composition. Early summer saw individual bands gathering in large camps that usually included the entire tribe.[21] The tribe came together once a year during the spring and summer to hold a large, community-based ceremony called the *okan* or Sun Dance. Bands would gather at an annual meeting place and, after the week-long ceremony was finished, the tribe would disperse back into bands to gather food and to hunt. Before reserves were created, the okan was traditionally the only time of year that all the tribes came together.

The social life of northwestern Plains people was structured further by societies.[22] Each tribe had a set of age-graded societies. Membership was based not on kinship but rather on age. An individual would therefore belong to several societies throughout his or her lifetime. Societies were essential to the survival of the entire tribe. They helped forge relationships and obligations with people beyond the immediate family and the band. Most important, societies were essential to the religious and physical well-being of communities.[23]

Within a given tribe, each society had roles and responsibilities that were both secular and religious.[24] Societies helped ensure the band's physical well-being by protecting it from temporal threats and by performing rituals intended to bring about good hunting and clear weather. Some societies had fixed rules, songs, and dances to perform; others owned medicine bundles and their associated rituals and powers; still others performed civil functions. For example, military societies or sodalities were responsible for fighting enemies but were also expected to perform internal policing tasks.[25] Other societies, such as the Horn Society, offered help, support, and spiritual guidance to members of the band.[26] The Horn Society was also in charge of deciding when the okan was to be held.

Most societies were strictly for men but, according to Siksika ceremonialist Reg Crowshoe, all members needed to have a female partner, usually a relative, in order to belong to a society. Some tribes had exclusively female societies – for example, the Old Women's Society, also known as the Motoki Society. The Motoki was a companion society to the Horn Society. The Motoki Society was responsible for acknowledging the importance of the buffalo and ensuring good luck in future hunts.[27] Aboriginal women also played important roles in other rituals and ceremonies, such as the okan, and many of them owned sacred bundles. Although information on women's ceremonial activities at the turn of the century is limited, what is available tells us that after the horse was introduced, male participation in ceremonial activities tended to be emphasized.[28]

Individuals received the power to heal and the rights to certain rituals and ceremonies through visions or dreams. Some dreams resulted in the creation of sacred objects called medicine bundles. A medicine bundle is a "generic term for any objects wrapped together and used for ritualistic purposes."[29] Individuals and societies could own medicine bundles, and bundles could be passed down, purchased, or sold. Other dreams or visions provided people with information on how to heal a particular illness through a spiritual helper. No two healers used the same medicine bundle, ritual, or ceremony, and these items thus remained the recipient's sole property unless sold.[30]

In Blackfoot, Nakoda, and Tsuu T'ina communities, healing rituals and ceremonies could either be conducted by individuals or they could involve entire groups or societies or even the entire tribe. One well-known community-based ceremony was the okan. This took place in the summer over seven days, was attended by all tribes, and was a composite of rituals and functions performed by individual ceremonialists.[31] During the year, an older woman made a vow to hold the okan, typically to aid in the recovery of a loved one. The Holy Woman's vow and the okan ensured the well-being of the tribe by fulfilling important social, religious, and political functions. The okan brought people together to restore and repair tribal unity. It also functioned as a means to re-establish balance with the environment when there were no buffalo or when there was ill health.[32]

The okan was the most important ceremony held by Plains people, one in which the Holy Woman played a central role. In preparation for it, the Holy Woman, with help from her husband, purchased a *natoas* (Sun Dance bundle),[33] performed the prescribed rituals, and acquired and dried the buffalo tongues used in the ceremony.[34] On the first day of the okan, the Holy Woman and her partner began a fast, which lasted for four days. On the fifth day, after the natoas was brought out and important rituals were performed, there was a procession to the Medicine Lodge, where the Centre Pole was raised. Inside the lodge the buffalo tongues were distributed. The first people to receive pieces of the dried tongues were the other virtuous women — those who had made vows to help loved ones. Afterwards, offerings were brought forward to be blessed by the sun to ensure future good luck. On the final day — after harmony was re-established and friendships and alliances were confirmed and renewed — the various bands left for their fall hunting grounds.

On balance, then, current scholarship agrees that the spiritual and religious practices of the northwestern Plains people were gendered, with women playing important and complementary roles to the more public and performative activities of men. The spiritual and communal well-being of communities has been well studied, but less attention has been paid to how Aboriginal peoples in southern Alberta addressed more mundane, day-to-day health concerns. The scholarly literature focuses on individual or collective responses to illness and ill health and says little about injuries, accidents, daily health and illness, and even life events such as childbirth and aging. When we turn our attention to the full range of healing work, we find possibilities for understanding how these societies responded to a wide array of health problems. For example, botanical cures were sometimes received in dreams, but more often than not plant knowledge was the result of an apprenticeship with an older woman in the community. Healers who used plants needed to know their seasonal availability and how to harvest, prepare, and administer them as medicine. Considerable expertise was required to properly use plant remedies. As a result, apprenticeships were long and often expensive, but they brought prestige. In the decades following the Second World War, ethnobotanist Joan Scott-Brown found that Nakoda women who wanted to learn about plants from their female elders had to purchase the knowledge. One woman interviewed by Scott-Brown expressed concern that because the learning process took a number of years and was expensive, her grandmother might pass away before she could afford to complete her education.[35] Turning our attention to these kinds of healing alternatives brings women's work to the fore.

The Siksika, Kainai, Piikani, Tsuu T'ina, and Nakoda, like many contemporary North American societies, practised a sexual division of labour that shaped women's use of space.[36] Women carried out most of their work in the camp, where they were responsible for setting up and looking after the lodge (which the women owned), raising children, tanning hides, making clothes and teepee covers, collecting roots and herbs, and preparing food.[37] Outside the camp, women's responsibilities included gathering edible and medicinal plants. In the early spring, women and children gathered wild plant foods, and in the late spring they dug bitterroot.[38] In July they dug wild prairie turnips and camass bulbs near the mountains. Midsummer saw women and children collecting savis berries, and they gathered chokecherries in October.[39] Besides their numerous gathering activities, women hunted and snared small game, fished, and helped their male counterparts with the buffalo hunt.[40] The men of the northwestern Plains often cut a striking image as they traversed the prairie on horseback.

Women's use of the terrain was less dramatic. Aboriginal women were more likely to be found picking berries in a patch or gathering herbs and roots in a grove of trees.[41] But because effective subsistence strategies were not always consistent with a strict sexual division of labour, there was some flexibility. Women's and men's activities were often determined by need and practicality. Gathering activities were often performed communally – in other words, men and children joined in.[42] As well, general knowledge about edible and medicinal plants was shared for the benefit of everyone. Plant gathering, much like a successful buffalo hunt, required the participation of the entire band.

There is considerable scholarly debate regarding the value placed on the labour of women and men in northwestern Plains communities, especially after European contact. Some have speculated that the introduction of horses, the robe trade, and European technology devalued women's work. The sources that support this argument are problematic because they were written mainly by non-Aboriginal men and coloured by the cultural values that Europeans placed on different types of work. As a result, the stereotype of the overworked Indian drudge has remained surprisingly resilient in white culture.

Nor was the performance of particular roles determined entirely by biological sex. Two-spirited – that is, cross-gendered – people were not unheard of in Plains societies. These people claimed an identity based on the performance of a social role rather than their physiology. Cross-gender women participated in activities typically relegated to men, such as raiding, and they sometimes took wives and had children. Other Aboriginal women were not cross-gender but played significant leadership roles and headed successful raiding parties.[43] The manly-hearted woman among the Blackfoot is yet another example of the complex ways in which gender operated among Aboriginal peoples. The manly-hearted woman was married, but she was also aggressive, independent, and ambitious and possessed sexual confidence.[44] To be manly-hearted was not necessarily to be cross-gendered; rather, it was a quality that allowed individual women to transgress certain gender norms and behaviours as they continued to be perceived as female.

There is evidence that these sorts of gender behaviours and social institutions persisted beyond the 1880s.[45] The degree to which Aboriginal women's status changed as a result of contact is difficult to determine. It is conceivable that the robe trade diminished the importance of certain aspects of women's work. Other possible causes are the decline of the fur trade, the establishment of reserves, and a decline in local resources. When examining so-called women's work, it is not the nature of that work that should be adjudicated but rather the cultural assumptions made about it. Feminist scholar Evelyn Blackwood contends that the performance of gender roles in Aboriginal communities should be regarded as the carrying out of a specific set of duties that were not inferior to but rather part of a "system of reciprocity that ensured the interdependence of the sexes."[46] The healing and caring work of Aboriginal women after the 1880s is an important window through which to trace not only cultural persistence but also important transformations in the meanings of women's work and knowledge.

Economic and Social Changes of the Nineteenth Century

The gendered organization of northwestern Plains peoples' social, cultural, and economic lives crystallized during the tremendous changes of the eighteenth and nineteenth centuries.[47] Between 1700 and 1730, the appearance of the horse and the gun set off a series of social and geopolitical shifts in Plains culture. In combination, the horse and the fur trade sparked what Bruce Trigger called in a different context a cultural florescence.[48] Because horses could travel longer distances and carry more material goods, they stimulated trade and communication.[49] Age-graded societies, medicine bundles, and the art of bead making all flourished. As mentioned earlier, however, there is still considerable scholarly debate about the impact of the horse and the expanding robe trade on the status and well-being of Plains women. Historian Andrew Isenberg argues that the horse created irreconcilable contradictions for Plains people because, as a symbol of wealth and success, it threatened communalism. Trade further complicated the situation by pushing Plains people toward commerce and individualism.[50] The introduction of the gun and the horse also shifted the balance of power on the northwestern Plains and brought about a long period of territorial conflict.[51] Indeed, the Blackfoot were almost constantly at war throughout these decades. They fought the Apsálooke (Crow), Shoshone, and Nez Perce to the south and southwest for horses and the Cree and Assiniboine to the north over hunting grounds.[52]

In the 1790s, contact between the Blackfoot and the Europeans increased with the establishment of trading posts – including Fort Edmonton and Rocky Mountain House – along the northern edges of Blackfoot territory. But the Blackfoot and Tsuu T'ina did not participate directly in the fur or robe trade until after the 1830s, when the American Fur Trade Company gained quick access to western trade routes along the Missouri River.[53] By the mid-nineteenth century, the Aboriginal peoples of the northwestern Plains were under a great deal of pressure from overhunting, European immigration, and the whisky trade. Shortages of buffalo developed as early as the 1830s. In some areas the scarcity of buffalo became a real concern by 1848.[54] A combination of overhunting and encroaching European settlement restricted seasonal subsistence activities. By the early 1880s, the buffalo had all but disappeared.

In addition to economic and territorial pressures, the people of the northwestern Plains faced a series of epidemics during the late eighteenth and nineteenth centuries. Using winter counts, Linea Sundstrom estimates that northern Plains groups suffered through thirty-six epidemics between 1714 and 1919.[55] The last pre-reserve smallpox epidemic endured by northwestern Plains groups was in 1869. An estimated 1,200 people of the Blackfoot Nation perished from it that year. Exposure to epidemics transformed Plains peoples' understanding of disease and contagion.[56] Human geographer Jody Decker maintains that, by 1869, Aboriginal people's awareness of contagion had "clearly changed and grown to include the concept of spreading an infectious disease through its victims and its discharges."[57] For example, when disease struck a mobile hunting and gathering band, its members practised their own form of quarantine by dispersing into small groups.

Women's knowledge of medicinal plants seems to have been a particularly important part of Aboriginal peoples' response to new health problems. Aboriginal healers adapted traditional remedies to treat the symptoms of new afflictions. When poor rations (including white bread and bad meat) caused digestive problems, Blackfoot women brewed a variety of herbal drinks to alleviate abdominal distress. Likewise, people with a tubercular cough were given infusions of yellow berries or tea made from willow. Willow bark, which contains salicin, the active ingredient in aspirin, helped soothe the patient.[58] The social and economic conditions that developed during the final decades of the nineteenth century, outlined in the following section, only increased the importance of healing and caregiving work performed by Siksika, Kainai, Piikani, Tsuu T'ina, and Nakoda women.

The Creation of Reserves

When Treaty 7 was negotiated in 1877, the inclusion of the Siksika, Kainai, Piikani, Tsuu T'ina, and Nakoda in one treaty had less to do with internal alliances and more to do with geographic proximity. At first, Treaty 7 was administered as a single agency under one Indian agent. By the late 1880s, however, the five tribes had been assigned their own communities and were managed separately. As an exception to this, the Tsuu T'ina and the Nakoda would remain part of the same agency until 1918. The treaty established an inequitable relationship between the federal government and Aboriginal peoples in southern Alberta. Perhaps even more significant, Treaty 7 reorganized the physical landscape of southern Alberta by separating Aboriginal space from white space. After the 1880s the movement of Aboriginal women between reserves and nearby settlements was restricted by authorities. It is therefore noteworthy that encounters between Aboriginal and white women persisted. Many of those encounters were premised on healing.

The federal government assigned the Siksika land east of Calgary, just south of the village of Cluny. Most of the reserve was open prairie with rolling hills and deep coulees. The region was subject to climate extremes – bitter cold and heavy snow in the winter, followed by severe drought with strong, dry winds and nightly frosts in the summer. The area was less than ideal for crops but quite suitable for grazing. Year after year, in his annual reports, the Blackfoot agent described his reserve's lack of agricultural success, except for potatoes. He blamed the failure on the poor climate. Limited water resources exacerbated the region's drought conditions. Small sloughs dotted the reserve landscape, but these dried up in the spring. Only two creeks contained water throughout the year: Arrowwood Creek in the reserve's southwest corner and Crowfoot Creek to the northeast.[59] In addition, the reserve lacked any significant timber: only cottonwood and poplar were found along the river.[60] The ability of the Siksika to build and maintain European-style houses was restricted by the shortage of water and timber, but rarely was this recognized.

The Kainai were at first offered land adjacent to the Siksika, but this tract of land was only four miles wide and located in one of the driest parts of Alberta. In 1883 the Kainai renegotiated the treaty and took land between the Belly and St. Mary rivers south of Fort Macleod. The negotiation made their reserve the largest in Canada.[61] Despite the reserve's size, it lacked timber, with the exception of clumps of berry shrubs at the north end and a few straggling cottonwoods in the valley. The Kainai faced much the same environmental challenges as the Siksika: their reserve's interior was dry, open, undulating plain without lakes or even ponds; the coulees were usually dry by early summer; and the temperature swings all but crippled the land for agriculture.[62]

The Piikani took land west of Fort Macleod. As with other parcels carved out for the Blackfoot Nation, the Piikani's land was most suitable for livestock grazing, even though the Department of Indian Affair's (DIA) intended to turn Aboriginal people into farmers. However, the Piikani were luckier that most groups with regard to the availability of timber. In the Porcupine Hills, they owned eleven-and-a-half acres of wood suitable for frame houses.[63] Thus, unlike the Siksika and the Kainai, the Piikani could build homes and barns without bankrupting themselves. Water for domestic purposes was obtained from the Oldman River, Beaver Creek, and Scott's Creek. These sources were, however, closed during the winter.[64]

Three Nakoda bands took land in the foothills west of Calgary near what had been the Morleyville mission. The Bow River ran through this reserve, fed by numerous streams and springs. Except for a small piece of land in the southeast, nearly all the reserve was gravelly and hilly and thus unsuitable for agriculture. This problem was exacerbated by high winds, drought, and early frosts.[65] The Nakoda pursued seasonal rounds of hunting in the mountains and worked as labourers for local ranchers because there was no opportunity for large-scale farming on their reserve.

After the signing of Treaty 7, the Tsuu T'ina settled on the Blackfoot Reserve. Then, after further negotiation, they acquired about seventy thousand acres of land located ten miles southwest of Fort Calgary in 1882.[66] As a result, the Tsuu T'ina Reserve today lies on the western outskirts of the expanding city of Calgary. Unlike the three tribes of the Blackfoot Nation, the Tsuu T'ina had greater access to water: a number of small streams that fed Fish Creek and the Elbow River crossed their land.[67] According to Indian agents at the Sarcee Reserve, a fairly large portion of the land on the eastern section of the reserve was suitable for cultivation, and the western section contained ample timber and firewood.[68] However, like the other reserves, the Sarcee Reserve faced environmental constraints on farming: drought, high winds, and frosts.[69] All three were typical of southern Alberta.

Treaty 7 did not immediately restrict the Aboriginal peoples of southern Alberta to their reserves. They continued to search for food and trading opportunities outside their reserve boundaries, and they would continue to do so until the 1880s.[70] During that decade the effects of the pass system and the growing presence of white settlers strained the capacity of Plains Aboriginal people to sustain their communities. By 1880 the bison had all but disappeared from western Canada – the last hunt in the northwestern United States was held in 1883.[71] The completion of the railway across the western prairies, the growth of ranching, and the Euro-Canadian settlement of southern Alberta further limited the ability of Aboriginal peoples to follow their old subsistence patterns. As a result, the residents of the Treaty 7 area increasingly turned to agriculture and ranching to try to support themselves.

Unfortunately, there would be very little successful agriculture in southern Alberta until extensive irrigation systems were built and dry-farming practices were perfected. During the early twentieth century, the Siksika, Kainai, Piikani, and Tsuu T'ina made strong efforts to dig irrigation ditches to make the land more fertile. The lack of water, however, continued to be a serious impediment. Even the Euro-Canadian settlers, who arrived in southern Alberta with a great deal of farming experience, found the lack of water a major obstacle and agriculture an expensive and high-risk venture.[72] Indeed, 40 percent of the non-Aboriginal homesteaders who tried to establish farms in southern Alberta between 1905 and 1930 failed to meet the government's conditions under the Dominion Lands Act.[73] It is noteworthy that while Indian agents often blamed crop failures on the unfavourable environment – that is, on the lack of timber or water – the same excuses were never offered for the inability of Aboriginal women to live up to the domestic standards set by Europeans. The shortage of water and building materials was rarely offered as an excuse for poor housekeeping.

Nation Building in Western Canada

After it purchased Rupert's Land from the Hudson's Bay Company in 1869, the newly founded Dominion of Canada took a series of steps to consolidate its control over the West and to open up lands for settlement. Key to all this was the Dominion Lands Act of 1872, which organized western settlement and determined how lands would be distributed. During the 1870s the seven western treaties were negotiated and signed with the region's Aboriginal peoples. In 1873 the North West Mounted Police (NWMP) was founded as a means to ensure peaceful and orderly Euro-Canadian settlement. Twelve years later, in 1885, the Canadian Pacific Railway was completed to carry settlers and manufactured products to western Canada and wheat back to the east.

These nation-building activities were accompanied by further measures designed to do more than restrict the original inhabitants to their reserves. New federal laws extended other forms of control over Aboriginal people. In 1876, as a first step, Ottawa consolidated all existing laws pertaining to Aboriginal peoples into one piece of legislation called the Indian Act. All future legislation affecting Aboriginal people would be based on this Act.[74] Later amendments to the Act were part of an attempt to control and transform land use, marriage and family structure, cultural beliefs and practices, and political participation among Aboriginal peoples.[75] One of the more coercive federal measures from that time was the pass system, a DIA policy introduced immediately after the 1885 Rebellion and never formally rescinded, which was designed to limit the mobility of Aboriginal peoples living on the Prairies.

This expansion of restrictive measures was accompanied by the development of the DIA bureaucracy. The department was created in 1880, and the minister of the Interior was placed in charge as the superintendent general. The department had two arms: the Land Sales Branch and the Accountant's Branch. Four new branches were created in 1885: the Statistics and School Branch (counting and education), the Correspondence Branch (communication), the Registry Branch (membership), and the Technical Branch (preparing surveys, drawings, and instructions). In 1889 a Land and Timber Branch was added to the department. These branches reflected the government's dual agenda, which was to manage Aboriginal people through services such as schools as it acquired their land and resources. As historians such as Douglas Leighton have shown, the DIA did not attract the best prospects for the civil service; as a result, most positions were filled by candidates who knew very little about Aboriginal people.[76]

The Health of the Siksika, Kainai, Piikani, Nakoda, and Tsuu T'ina, 1880-1930

Aboriginal people responded as well as they could to the new challenges they faced from Euro-Canadian settlement. Poverty and severe malnutrition during the 1880s exacerbated the impact of European diseases. Historian John Ewers estimates that in Montana between 1882 and 1885, of 7,000 Piikani, somewhere between 250 and 550 starved to death.[77] Ethnographer George Bird Grinnell, who lived among the Piikani during the 1880s, placed this number much higher. He calculated that 2,500 people (about one-third of the population) had starved to death.[78] The situation in southern Alberta was not much better. After spending the winter of 1880-81 hunting in Montana, hundreds of starving Blackfoot crossed the border into Canada. Norman Thomas Macleod, the brother of Colonel James Macleod and newly appointed Indian agent for all of Treaty 7, made efforts to feed the seven thousand hungry Aboriginal people who then occupied southern Alberta. The federal government responded by ordering Macleod to reduce rations. Macleod resigned in disgust in 1882.[79] The reports of starvation were not addressed seriously by the federal government, despite the pleas of individual Indian agents and other government employees.[80]

During the late 1870s and early 1880s, the total population of the Siksika, Kainai, Piikani, Nakoda, and Tsuu T'ina who lived in Alberta was around seven thousand. On Treaty 7 reserves, morbidity and mortality rates remained high throughout the late nineteenth and early twentieth centuries.[81] At the Sarcee Reserve, in 1887, for example, Inspector Alex McGibbon reported six births and seventeen deaths – one family alone had lost three children to tuberculosis.[82] These high death rates did not continue throughout the period of this study; even so, by 1918 the Aboriginal population of Treaty 7 had declined by more than half, to just under three thousand people.[83]

Recurrences of contagious diseases such as smallpox, whooping cough, and measles decreased but did not disappear entirely. For instance, a major smallpox epidemic struck every Aboriginal community in southern Alberta in 1904. That year, the death rate at the Blackfoot Reserve was 100 per 1,000, while at the Blood Reserve it was 110 per 1,000.[84] Epidemics were not the only serious concern. By the 1890s, diseases of poverty such as tuberculosis had become a source of misery for Treaty 7 people. By the turn of the century, TB rates for prairie Aboriginal peoples were 42.6 per 1000 – nearly twenty times the rate for non-Aboriginal Canadians.[85] Economic disruption and inadequate rations had left Aboriginal people ill-equipped to deal with chronic and often fatal infections.

Historians have thoroughly documented that the federal government was unwilling to make the necessary commitments to deal with the social and economic dislocations experienced by Aboriginal peoples at the end of the nineteenth century and the beginning of the twentieth.[86] Maureen Lux, in *Medicine That Walks,* describes the impact of substandard rations, hunger, ragged clothing, and torn lodges on the health of Aboriginal communities. In the Treaty 7 area, inadequate housing was an especially severe problem because of the scarcity of building timber. The Siksika in particular faced an acute housing shortage throughout most of the period discussed in this book.[87] Similarly, Hugh Shewell, in *Enough to Keep Them Alive,* describes Ottawa's parsimony in response to requests for social assistance. Aboriginal people were primary targets of the federal government's persistent efforts to practise fiscal constraint.[88]

Poor living conditions remained the greatest challenge in attempts to address the ill health of Aboriginal people. Throughout the twentieth century, the health of Aboriginal peoples in southern Alberta was negatively affected by terrible living conditions and social and economic confusion. These circumstances exacerbated illnesses of poverty, including tuberculosis. Between 1891 and 1900, 199 deaths were recorded among the Tsuu T'ina; 46 percent of them were TB related.[89] A study conducted by the Canadian Tuberculosis Association in 1924 revealed that although Aboriginal peoples constituted only 4.5 percent of Canada's population, they accounted for 25 percent of all deaths from TB – a staggering proportion.[90]

Little would be done to improve this situation until after the Second World War. During the Great Depression of the 1930s, federal spending on Aboriginal peoples dwindled, especially with respect to medical services. The DIA's annual report for 1933 indicated that the federal government had provided 20 percent less money for medical services than the preceding year. With regard to TB, the report stated that "no progress can now be made toward the solution of the tuberculosis problem. On the contrary the department has been forced to refuse the admission to sanatorium of many cases which the attending physician indicated would improve under proper care."[91]

Medical historians maintain that improvements in living conditions and diet during the early twentieth century had a greater impact on the health of North Americans than the advent of scientific medicine. They point, for example, to Herbert Ames's 1897 study of Montreal, which documented how death rates fluctuated dramatically among neighbourhoods.[92] For example, the death rate for Montreal as a whole in 1895 was 24.81 per 1,000, yet the death rates (from 32.32 to 35.51 per 1000) were much higher in working-class wards that were predominantly French Canadian.[93] This historiographical emphasis on the effects of living standards has influenced Lux's examination of material conditions in Aboriginal communities in western Canada. She has shown that the standard of living for Aboriginal people remained well below that of the average Euro-Canadian into the 1930s and 1940s.[94]

Faced with this demographic and economic crisis, the federal government had little choice but to offer health services to Aboriginal people. When the DIA was first created, it took no formal steps to provide medical services to those in its charge. The BNA Act stated that medical services were a provincial jurisdiction and that federal authority over medical matters was limited to immigrant health and quarantine practices. As a result, any medical services made available by the DIA were piecemeal. They were often initiated only in response to requests from concerned Indian agents, missionaries, and settlers. For instance, the DIA hired the NWMP surgeon after 1877 to enforce vaccination and quarantine.[95] In 1883 physicians from settlements adjacent to Treaty 7 reserves replaced the NWMP surgeon. These medical officers were expected to attend Aboriginal people in their homes and camps and to oversee residential and day schools. The doctors visited the reserves once a month and were on call for emergencies. These part-time physicians were the extent of medical services provided to Aboriginal people by the DIA. Although Aboriginal peoples were considered the federal government's responsibility (in other words, ineligible for municipal or provincial services), the DIA continued to drag its feet when it came to providing them with health care.

In the 1890s the churches and their missionary organizations began to develop a broader system of medical services for Aboriginal people. Anglican, Methodist, and Roman Catholic groups established hospitals, school infirmaries, and dispensaries to address ill health among their Aboriginal congregations. By this time, missions and missionaries had been informally providing Aboriginal people with basic medical aid and nursing care for several decades. These developments mirrored those in Euro-Canadian communities in southern Alberta that were large enough to support a medical doctor. On reserves where the local mission was unable to erect a hospital, Euro-Canadian women served as both matrons and nurses in the residential schools. The churches and their missions tried to provide some medical and nursing care for the reserves in their charge. Department of Indian Affairs medical officers continued to make monthly visits, and they included the church-run hospitals as part of their rounds. The DIA contributed little funding for these institutions. It was not until 1904, when the position of medical inspector was created, that the DIA began to take a more active role in Aboriginal health care.[96] Between 1900 and 1920, the DIA provided public health nurses for schools and temporary nursing stations, but only when it decided that conditions required them. During the 1920s and 1930s, the DIA took over management of the Blackfoot and Blood hospitals and built medical facilities at the Stoney, Sarcee, and Peigan reserves. Besides taking a more direct role in hospital management, the DIA created public health programs to deal with what the department believed were the underlying causes of ill health on reserves. A public health service was finally created in 1904, and a travelling nurse program was instituted in 1922. This system was formalized as the DIA's Indian Health Services in 1927.

Conclusion

The enormous social, political, and economic transformations taking place in the late nineteenth and early twentieth centuries altered the landscape of southern Alberta, and it was during these decades that reserves took on real physical and social meanings. Nevertheless, Aboriginal and newcomer women continued to encounter one another. They first met in the houses and sod huts of Euro-Canadian women and later in the tents, camps, and houses of Aboriginal women. As the West underwent more Euro-Canadian settlement, fewer newcomers drew from the therapeutic knowledge of Aboriginal women. Simultaneously, the healing encounters between Aboriginal and Euro-Canadian women became more formal, more often than not taking place in institutional space. In some situations, depending on the type of illness and the quality of service, Aboriginal women drew from the medical services of Euro-Canadian women; in other situations, they continued to rely on traditional knowledge acquired over generations. Although less visible, Aboriginal women possessed significant knowledge about the medicinal nature of local plants and applied them on a daily basis for the good of the community. The decline in missionary women's use of Aboriginal women's healing expertise fundamentally altered relations between them. Aboriginal women were not unaware that the help of Euro-Canadian women came attached with conditions; therefore, they were constantly negotiating when and how to use Western medicine. The following chapters outline this slow and uneven process.

2

Setting the Stage

Engendering the Therapeutic Culture of the Siksika, Kainai, Piikani, Tsuu T'ina, and Nakoda

The roles of women and men in northwestern Plains cultures were mediated by cultural understandings of gender. As the previous chapter shows, women and men performed separate but complementary tasks in their communities. The activities of women centred on the camp. Women were responsible for setting up and maintaining the lodge, gathering roots and herbs, preparing food, caring for children, tanning hides, and making clothing and teepee covers. Men were in charge of hunting large game, protecting the camp, looking after the horses, and raiding. Although most scholars acknowledge this functional division of labour in the culture of northwestern Plains people, few recognize the gender-specific nature of Aboriginal curative and caregiving practices. Aboriginal women were responsible for a particular set of healing skills within the therapeutic repertoire of northwestern Plains people. Much of the day-to-day curative and nursing labour was performed by women. Medicinal plant use and midwifery were part of an intergenerational tradition of female-centred knowledge, yet this uniquely female skill set has been largely unexplored. More visible and masculine aspects of northwestern Plains culture, such as the buffalo hunt and the medicine man, have received far more attention from scholars and European audiences. The private nature of women's work and the predominance of white male observers at the turn of the nineteenth century has coloured popular European views about the healing practices of northwestern Plains people.

There are several reasons why the therapeutic labour of northwestern Plains women was overlooked by Europeans during the late nineteenth and early twentieth centuries. First, a great deal of women's healing work took place in private and was not as visible as more public activities such as the buffalo hunt. Nor were women's everyday curative tasks as visually spectacular and eye-catching as the spiritual and exotic components of northwestern Plains medicine. Public healing rituals and ceremonies such as efforts to control the weather – which was most often performed by men – drew far greater attention than the banalities of childbirth and family illnesses. Second, most people who observed and published about northwestern Plains culture during this period were male – missionaries, fur traders, naturalists, government employees, ethnographers, and anthropologists. These men came west, fleeing the pressures of urbanization and industrialization, for the opportunity to experience the excitement and thrill of the last "untouched" North American "frontier." For many of them, an essential part of this journey was documenting what they believed to be the final vestiges of a noble if vanishing race.[1]

These amateur ethnographers and anthropologists generally focused on gathering the recollections of elderly Aboriginal people, who described for them the so-called traditional culture of northwestern Plains people. These amateurs were fascinated by descriptions of Aboriginal medicine, and they tended to focus on its supernatural elements. As a consequence, Aboriginal medicine was largely depicted as rituals – performed primarily by men – that involved communing with the spiritual *and* material worlds. The inordinate attention paid to such practices in these observers' articles and monographs profoundly shaped European perceptions of northwestern Plains culture.

The dialogue between these ethnographers and the people they studied was not entirely one-sided. Many European observers spent long periods of time in Aboriginal communities. These contacts could be intimate and prolonged. In some cases vital cultural information was passed on to the visitor only after he had become a member of the family. Information about medicine bundles would therefore be revealed only after he had been adopted into the family, society, or tribe.[2] In other instances Aboriginal leaders asked ethnographers and anthropologists to intercede on their people's behalf with the federal government. In the United States, for example, the Blackfeet asked amateur anthropologist and naturalist George Bird Grinnell to use his political connections in New York and Washington to influence Indian policy.[3] Although sympathetic – indeed, even critical of particular Indian agents – Grinnell never questioned the fundamental objective of Indian policy: assimilation.

This request made to Grinnell tells us that Aboriginal people were not passive participants in ethnographic encounters. In other words, there was an exchange – albeit an unequal one – between the observers and the people they were observing. As they recorded northwestern Plains culture, ethnographers and anthropologists were made aware of the social, economic, and political problems faced by Aboriginal people. As a result, whatever private agendas these observers harboured, many of them did document Aboriginal peoples' contemporary concerns and social practices. The portrait of the northwestern Plains people produced by European observers in the late nineteenth century was not simplistic. According to historian Sherry Smith, it "asserted Indians' humanity, artistry, community, and spirituality."[4]

Nineteenth-century ethnographers and anthropologists tended to declare that Aboriginal people were a vanishing race. This coloured their accounts of Aboriginal history, economics, social organization, politics, and belief systems. Early observers' accounts of Aboriginal plant use and curative regimes are most important for this study. Their texts suggest that northwestern Plains women played an important role in healing. Knowledge of medicinal plants, expertise in midwifery, and skill at mechanical healing (e.g., the setting of bones) were important to northwestern Plains communities, and Aboriginal women played a prominent role in all three.

Ethnographers and Anthropologists

At the same time that Aboriginal peoples in the West were undergoing a transformation in their lifeways, the discipline of anthropology was changing in profound ways. In the 1870s and 1880s, anthropology was evolving from an amateurs' pastime into a university-based discipline with claims to professionalism and scientific objectivity. George Bird Grinnell,[5] James Willard Schultz,[6] John Maclean,[7] and Walter McClintock[8] were among the amateur ethnographers and anthropologists who studied the Blackfoot during the 1880s and 1890s.[9] None of these authors possessed formal or scholarly training, yet their knowledge and observations about Aboriginal people were readily accepted by the general public, by scholarly institutions, and by the government because they built on a long tradition of colonial travel writing, for which there existed a strong popular demand.[10]

Clark Wissler, one of the first university-educated anthropologists to conduct fieldwork among the Blackfoot, was among this group. In the late 1890s, he studied under Franz Boas, the man who almost single-handedly trained the first cohort of American anthropologists. In 1902 Boas hired Wissler as his assistant at the American Museum of Natural History.[11] In 1903 he sent Wissler to do fieldwork among the Dakota. When Boas resigned from the museum in 1905, Wissler replaced him as curator of ethnology. In 1907 Wissler became the curator of the Anthropology Department, a post he held until his retirement in 1942.[12]

Wissler began his fieldwork among the Blackfeet in 1908. He relied heavily on David Duvall, whose father was French Canadian and whose mother was Piikani. Wissler had met Duvall in 1903, in Browning, Montana, the Blackfeet Reservation's agency town.[13] Duvall interviewed Blackfeet informants and collected materials for Wissler until his death by suicide in 1911.[14] Quite probably, Duvall's insider status is what enabled him to record information that anthropologists and ethnographers could not.[15] Through Duvall and his female relatives, Wissler gained access to information that otherwise would have been closed to him.

ETHNOGRAPHICAL AND ANTHROPOLOGICAL DEFINITIONS OF MEDICINE

In the accounts of the early ethnographers and anthropologists, we encounter more than one definition of Aboriginal medicine. This is apparent when we examine their writings to glean northwestern Plains peoples' understandings of health and illness. These works do not reflect any clear consensus about what medicine meant in the culture they were recording. In his article "Blackfoot Medical Priesthood," which was published in 1909, John Maclean writes that medicine men performed many duties: they cured diseases with medicines, hypnotism, and incantations; they dispelled evil spirits by exorcism; they acted as prophets and predicted future weather and game movements; and they practised necromancy.[16] Walter McClintock defined the practitioner as "more of a magician than a medical doctor. His vocation is to instruct and guide in the avoidance of acts that are 'bad medicine' and therefore unlucky."[17] He described the work of a medicine man as "performing mysterious ceremonies, or using other approved means for controlling the supernatural powers and averting the malevolence of evil spirits."[18] In *Blackfoot Lodge Tales,* George Bird Grinnell wrote that Blackfeet doctors were called *I-so-kin'-uh-kin* (loosely translated, "heavy singer for the sick") because "all doctors sing while endeavouring to work their cures."[19] All of these observers did agree, however, that medicine men shared one common trait: the ability to deal in some way with the spiritual or supernatural.

According to these observers, medicine men filled multiple roles: priest, healer, medium, necromancer. They were also aware that European understandings of Blackfoot medicine were limited.[20] Wissler and Grinnell regarded language as the greatest barrier to understanding. Maclean and McClintock contended that it was the lack of Christianity among Aboriginal peoples that compelled them to believe in what Maclean referred to as medicine beliefs.[21] These observers allowed that medicine men did perform a curative role, but rarely did they outline it in any detail.

This fascination with the supernatural and the exotic did not prevent ethnographers and anthropologists from recording observations about medicinal plants and the so-called mechanical aspects of healing. What these observers did *not* do was discuss healing in ways that treated the supernatural and the physical as parts of a single system. They instead understood the two as separate realms. Kainai elder Rufus Goodstriker highlighted the differences between European and Aboriginal concepts of healing in an interview in 1983. White doctors "split the body in three ways, body, mind, and spirit. In the Indian way, it is the opposite. Spirit, mind, and body. Everything is connected."[22]

Several substantive observations can be made from these early texts. First, they highlight the more visible and exotic aspects of northwestern Plains peoples' curative practices. Indeed, when writing about the causes of illness and the methods used for healing, these observers most often placed their accounts alongside those of myths and legends. They also emphasized the spectacle of particular rituals. For example, in the *Old North Trail*, McClintock relates the origins of the Thunder Medicine Pipe and bundle: "The medicine pipe was given to the Blackfeet long ago, when the Thunder struck down a man. While he lay on the ground, the thunder Chief appeared in a vision, showing him a pipe, and saying, 'I have chosen you that I might give you this pipe ... Gather together also a medicine bundle, containing the skins of the many animals and birds, which go with it. Whenever any of your people are sick, or dying, a vow must be made and a ceremonial given with a feast. The sick will then be restored to health.'"[23] These observers did not discuss the symptoms of illnesses, the different plants to treat them, or who prepared and administered those treatments. One possible reason for this oversight could be that, because they were men, they were not granted access to more intimate details of day-to-day healing practices.

The substantive therapeutic skills of medicine men were overlooked in favour of recording spectacle. A common set of highly formulaic descriptions can be found in the texts of early ethnographers and anthropologists, who shared many of the same conventions when they wrote about how Aboriginal people acquired their healing powers. These accounts often note the presence of a non-human or other worldly agent and describe how knowledge – how to construct and use a bundle, how to perform a ritual, or how to use plants – most often came in a dream.[24] Descriptions of healing skills that relied on knowledge passed down through the generations from mother to daughter or from elder to apprentice are remarkably absent in these texts.

Accounts of healing ceremonies likewise focused on sensory elements: singing, praying, dancing, smoking sweetgrass, using medicine bundles, and following the rules that govern particular ceremonies. McClintock describes a healing ceremony: "The medicine men chanted and prayed all night and day. When one was exhausted another took his place. Their powers to heal came from the otter, the grizzly, the mink, and the buffalo. Each drummed in turn, imitating the movements of the animal he represented ... The sick man was brought back to life three times by rubbing his body with sacred paint and holding the medicine pipe before his face."[25] Whether describing the acquisition of healing powers or the conduct of healing ceremonies, these authors stressed the fantastic and almost impossible and left out the demonstrable impact of Aboriginal healing practices on specific symptoms or illnesses.

Two elements of these descriptions are immediately obvious. First, the healing practices of the northwest Plains people were not placed in their proper context. By focusing on the more public and exotic aspects of their curative practices, anthropologists and ethnographers emphasized only one facet of Aboriginal medicine. Cures intended to deal with particular physical symptoms such as coughs, sore throats, indigestion, and headaches were not recorded in any detail. A similar observation has been made regarding the cultural practices of other Aboriginal groups. For example, Michael Angel's examination of the Ojibwa's *midewiwin* ceremony found that most European accounts referred only to a single aspect of the ceremony – one that the observer was especially impressed with.[26] These observers described only the public and spectacular aspects of Aboriginal health care, as if they were the sum of Aboriginal medicine. They failed to notice that these aspects were but one part of a broader set of beliefs and practices intended to serve important social, religious, and healing functions.[27]

Second, this focus on the exotic cast a veil over the historical record and ignored Aboriginal women's deep knowledge of medicinal plants and their uses. Aboriginal women's day-to-day healing mostly involved family illnesses and accidents. Nursing and caregiving took place in private space, outside the gaze of male non-Aboriginal observers. As a consequence, it went unobserved. Because home care was normal practice for many European–North Americans before the early twentieth century – that is, nothing out of the ordinary to Aboriginal *or* non-Aboriginal people – it was perceived as not worth recording.

Medicinal Plant Use

Ethnographers and anthropologists did however observe some things about Plains people's healing practices. For example, in *Blackfoot Lodge Tales,* Grinnell records that various herbs or roots were boiled and then made into lotions or poultices to treat ulcers, boils, and sprains and that rheumatism was treated either by the sweat lodge or the application of hot rocks or by inserting thorns into the flesh and setting fire to them. He also describes a yellow fungus that the Blackfeet used as a purgative. They gathered it from pine trees, dried and pulverized it, and administered it dry or in an infusion.[28] These observations often involved the observer's own illness. For instance, Schultz writes that when he was sick with a fever, Yellow Wolf's wife gave him sweet sage tea.[29]

The most extensive description of Aboriginal plant use during this period comes from McClintock, who lists more than sixty different plants used by the Piikani for food and medicinal and spiritual purposes. He provides this botanical information in an Appendix to the *Old North Trail*.[30] According to the Appendix, plants were used to treat fevers, swellings, stomach aches, weight gain, sore throats, cramps, headaches, heartburn, hemorrhaging, diarrhea, and so on. Sandra Leslie Peacock notes that McClintock's study is to this day highly regarded by Piikani elders.[31]

McClintock's interest in the plants used by the Blackfeet was unusual for his time, and his attention to detail was painstaking. His notes detail how and when plants were harvested, prepared, and applied as remedies. He was remarkable not only for his interest but also for his efforts to seek out Piikani women who would teach him. He records that it was Blackfeet women who maintained their culture's knowledge of medicinal and food plants.[32] It was they who told him these plants' local names and explained their various uses.[33] His observations are supported by later interviews with Kainai elders. Rufus Goodstriker revealed that it was his mother who had taught him how to use herbs to heal people.[34] In a comparable cultural context, Marion Carrier, a Cree elder, stated that it had been her grandmother who taught her everything when she went to live with her.[35]

McClintock likewise observed the sexual division of labour in northwestern Plains society and commented on the different roles performed by women and men. Women were generally responsible for collecting vegetable material and, according to McClintock, they permitted no interference from men, "who were naturally unfit for such tasks, because they lacked the requisite knowledge and training."[36] Perhaps the participation of Aboriginal men in gathering activities was a later result of settlement on reserves. Until recently, Aboriginal women's food-gathering activities have been characterized as merely supplementing a diet in which buffalo meat predominated. Archaeologist Sandra Peacock refers to this oversight as the "tyranny of the ethnographic record."[37] That record has largely ignored the importance of plants and the work of Aboriginal women in the subsistence activities of northwestern Plains people. In her examination of Piikani ethnobotany, Peacock notes the failure of anthropologists and ethnographers to record information regarding vegetable material and its uses. Two possible reasons can be offered for this oversight. The first is that vegetable material has not been preserved in the archaeological record. Conversely, the northwestern Plains are littered with buffalo bones. The second relates to the gender of early ethnographers and anthropologists: as white men, these observers likely had very little access to or interest in the less public activities of Aboriginal women.[38] Feminist ethnobotanist Joan Scott-Brown's recent work confirms this oversight. In a study of plant use among Nakoda women undertaken in the 1970s, Scott-Brown restricted her fieldwork to women because it was the community's medicine women who dispensed botanical remedies and who passed on their healing expertise and knowledge to other women.[39] Nakoda women knew where to find the important plants and roots and how to concoct and administer treatments.

Accordingly, accepted wisdom holds that the buffalo provided northwestern Plains people with everything they needed. Grinnell's influential work on the Kainai, for example, provides a very brief description of the plants they ate but devotes an entire chapter to hunting.[40] Anthropologist Oscar Lewis, in an unpublished paper on Kainai economics written in 1942, remarks that "the buffalo hunt was probably the most important economic activity" for the Kainai.[41] Since the turn of the nineteenth century, the Aboriginal peoples of the northwestern Plains have epitomized the so-called Indian for most Europeans.[42] Images of the buffalo hunter, the warrior, and the chief have proven especially potent and enduring.[43] Patricia Albers, in her 1983 study of Plains women, contends that the side of Plains Indian life most often conjured by the public is "the male half, which is a universe dominated by diplomacy, warfare, and hunting" – a habit of mind that until relatively recently had a parallel in non-Aboriginal history.[44]

When northwestern Plains women do appear in the historical record, they are depicted in a very negative light. They are either described as beasts of burden, or – as in the reserve period – they are condemned for their supposedly poor housekeeping skills and lascivious natures.[45] Recent feminist scholarship has responded to the omission of Aboriginal women in the historical record. It has shown that Aboriginal women played essential roles in the mobile economy of the northwestern Plains people through their knowledge, collection, and use of wild plants. Indeed, the ripening and availability of wild plants used for food and medicine often determined camp movements, and these subsistence activities were a core part of Aboriginal survival strategies.[46] We can only glimpse this complex female economy in anthropological sources. To see it whole, we must listen for the silences and then fill them with other forms of evidence.

Midwifery

Another area of medicine that Aboriginal women were responsible for was midwifery. Indeed, midwifery in Aboriginal society underscores the sexual division of labour that differentiated many Aboriginal healing activities in northwestern Plains communities. Midwifery also draws attention to the female-male divide that shaped the venues to which male European observers had access during this period. Healing skills that focused on the female body were hardly mentioned in the texts of these observers. Not until the late 1930s, when female anthropologists began conducting fieldwork and interviewing Aboriginal women, was a range of midwifery activities recorded (see Chapter 6).

Discussions about childbirth in northwestern Plains culture are almost entirely absent from the texts of early ethnographers and anthropologists. This oversight is especially noteworthy because Blackfoot midwifery practices incorporated many of the same conventions that observers found so enthralling in other healing ceremonies, such as the use of knowledge derived from dreams; the use of medicine bundles; certain proscriptive taboos; singing, praying, and dancing; and the smoking of sweetgrass. Yet however preoccupied these early observers (and later historians) were with what they viewed as exotic rituals, they did not record anything about midwifery, even though it was an important aspect of Aboriginal healing practices. In part this is because men were not welcome during the birthing process. Aboriginal women were attended by midwives and by experienced female family members and friends.

An exception is the work of Wissler and his field assistant Duvall. As an insider, Duvall was able to provide rare but significant descriptions of childbirth in Aboriginal communities. In his 1912 publication the *Social Organization and Ritualistic Ceremonies of the Blackfoot Indians*, Wissler (with Duvall's assistance) describes what Aboriginal women did when they were about to give birth: "They retire to an isolated tipi where they are attended by other women, men not being admitted. A medicine woman may be called, who usually administers decoctions for internal use, supposed to facilitate delivery. For bearing down, the patient holds to a pole of the tipi, an attendant grasping her around the waist. When delivered she is laced up with a piece of skin or rawhide as support. She is then required to walk or creep about the tipi for a while instead of resting quietly, in the belief that recovery will be hastened thereby."[47]

It is unlikely that Wissler ever witnessed an actual birth because he did not conduct his own fieldwork. Indeed, men were prohibited from approaching the birthing place. Only the father was welcome, and even his presence posed some risk.[48] It is likely that Duvall gathered this material from his female kin. And it is significant that Wissler's account provides only general information about childbirth and proscriptive taboos. Duvall was Aboriginal, and this knowledge would have been easy for him to acquire through female relatives or friends.

In his writing Wissler does not include detailed descriptions of the actual midwifery skills of midwives or of the plants they used. Instead, he describes the taboos and rituals that Aboriginal women observed during labour – such as the sorts of clothing or jewellery they were supposed to wear during childbirth, how a pregnant woman should be approached, and who was allowed to attend the mother during labour – and certain beliefs regarding the significance of birthmarks, twins, and stillborn babies.[49] More detailed descriptions of Aboriginal midwifery practices are more recent. In part this is a result of Aboriginal people trying to reclaim authority over the birth process, including the gender and race of the observers. In part it is a function of women's efforts to de-medicalize childbirth by looking to Aboriginal culture as a model.

Conclusion

Modern-day studies in ethnobotany have catalogued the botanical knowledge central to the healing cultures of Treaty 7 people and have documented the gendered nature of that knowledge. Southern Alberta's Aboriginal women used their expertise in local plant resources to address health, illness, injury, and problems in pregnancy and childbirth. This chapter uses historical sources to demonstrate the existence of these practices in the late nineteenth and early twentieth centuries, along with the ways in which medicinal plant use built on the sexual division of labour in Aboriginal society. The partial and incomplete evidence in anthropological texts reminds us that – however great the observers' emphasis on exotic, dramatic, and masculine healing rituals – Aboriginal women also made important contributions to the health of their communities. As McClintock and Wissler documented clearly, women's botanical knowledge and midwifery skills were still in place in the 1880s. The next chapter reveals that these skills were shared with Euro-Canadian settlers as they began to arrive in southern Alberta in the 1880s.

3
Giving Birth
Women's Health Work and Western Settlement, 1850-1900

In the 1850s, fur traders, missionaries, the North West Mounted Police (NWMP), and settlers began arriving in the West in rapidly increasing numbers, and they came to rely on Aboriginal women for a range of curative services. The healing and nursing skills applied by Aboriginal women in their own communities became an important resource for non-Aboriginal people, especially women. Serious illnesses and accidents were common among newcomers to western Canada, where people lived and worked in a harsh environment far from established support networks. The presence of women guaranteed the need for expertise and experience in pregnancy, childbirth, and childhood illnesses. In the absence of traditional familial systems of care and Western doctors, nurses, and medical facilities, the informal health work performed by Aboriginal women among newcomers created a space in which people came into contact with one another across the divides of race and culture.

Until recently, histories of western Canada have neglected the vital role that Aboriginal women performed in settler communities from the latter half of the nineteenth century and into the early twentieth. Historian Sarah Carter regards this historical amnesia as part of the insidious process of colonization. At the turn of the century, highly specific meanings were attached to the culturally constructed categories of Aboriginal and white women. Tracing public discourse after 1885, Carter found that white women were characterized in newspapers and travel literature as harbingers of civilization. Conversely, Aboriginal women, when not entirely absent from the landscape of western Canada, were increasingly represented as dangerous and immoral.[1] These representations were used to legitimate the segregation and marginalization of Aboriginal peoples. Although they are important to acknowledge, these representations say very little about the day-to-day experiences of women.

A reassessment of the twinned processes of settlement and colonialism reveals a much more complicated portrait of contact between Aboriginal and non-Aboriginal people during this period. The life of the average white woman living on a western ranch or farm was very different from the "fragile, rarefied, genteel, 'civilizer' ideal."[2] Settler women worked terribly hard as they ran the homestead and cared for children. They were often left alone without the aid of other adults for long stretches of time while their husbands, fathers, or brothers worked elsewhere.[3] Thus, when women gave birth, were sick, or simply required help, their male relatives were often absent. As a result, accounts of Aboriginal women coming to the aid of white settler women are a common refrain in stories related by settlers years later. Aboriginal women worked as midwives, healers, and caregivers for white settlers in a region where newcomers did not have extended familial networks or access to Western doctors, nurses, and hospitals.

After 1900 the number of non-Aboriginal people in the West grew dramatically. The population of western Canada increased from roughly 400,000 in 1901 to 2.4 million in 1931.[4] The settlement in southern Alberta occurred at a slightly slower pace than in Saskatchewan and central Alberta. The Palliser Expedition in the late 1850s had concluded that the climate of southwestern Alberta was too dry for farming. This deterred early large-scale white settlement, but not the Department of Indian Affairs' efforts to transform Treaty 7 reserves into agricultural paradises.

In 1881 the total non-Aboriginal population of the North-West Territories (present-day Saskatchewan and Alberta) was only 6,974.[5] Even after the railway through Alberta was completed in 1883, there was no great rush of settlers and farmers to the southern part of the province.[6] Mining towns developed after 1874, and the rest of the region was dedicated to ranching, which emerged as a major industry in the 1880s and 1890s. Ranchers were reluctant to have farmers infringe on their grazing lands, and extensive tracts were held by the Hudson's Bay Company, the Canadian Pacific Railway (CPR), and the colonization companies. The largest group to come to southern Alberta during this period were the Mormons, who arrived in the late 1880s and 1890s.[7] They established farms around present-day

Cardston. Between 1896 and the First World War, Alberta – its agricultural land in particular – came to be seen as the "last best West." After 1896 the settler population began to increase until non-Aboriginal people dramatically outnumbered Aboriginal people. According to the census, the Province of Alberta had a population of 65,876 in 1901, of whom only 5,620 were Aboriginal.[8] After that year, so many settlers flooded Alberta that half of Alberta's residents were born outside Canada until the 1930s.[9] Alberta had a population of 588,454 in 1921; one decade later, that number had increased to 731,605.[10]

As the population increased, ranching declined in importance until, by 1912, farming had become the biggest industry in southern Alberta. One driver for this was irrigation projects. Another was innovations in dry-farming practices.[11] In 1901 Alberta had only one city, Calgary, with a population of 4,091.[12] After 1901 the province experienced substantial urban growth and economic diversification. By 1905, Edmonton and Calgary, strategically located along railway lines, had emerged as the new province's urban centres. The combined population of Calgary and Edmonton was 30,119 – one-third of the provincial total in 1906.[13] By 1921 the population of those two cities had grown fourfold to nearly 120,000, but small towns and farming communities were growing at an even faster rate. Calgary and Edmonton represented only one-fifth of the province's population. Both cities relied heavily on the agricultural hinterland, serving as distribution and processing centres for agricultural products. Regional centres such as Lethbridge and Medicine Hat serviced the Treaty 7 communities of southern Alberta. So too did much smaller towns such as Fort Macleod, Taber, and Cardston.[14] The resource economy of southern Alberta began to diversify, especially during the boom years of the mid-1920s, to include sugar beets, petroleum, and coal. Then the province was hit hard by the Great Depression.

This dramatic population growth and urbanization led to corresponding developments in infrastructure, such as hospitals staffed by doctors and nurses. The founding of these eroded the need for non-Aboriginal people to make use of Aboriginal women's healing skills. This process was not, however, uniform. Geography, class, race, and ethnicity shaped non-Aboriginal people's use of and access to the healing expertise of Aboriginal women. Even though the healing knowledge and work of Aboriginal women was obscured by the arrival of Western medical practitioners, Aboriginal women continued to play essential therapeutic roles in both Aboriginal and settler communities.

Aboriginal Women and Newcomers, 1850-1900

In the late nineteenth century, dramatic new advances in scientific knowledge were revolutionizing Western medical practices. Yet until 1900 – for some people, much longer – modern medical care was often beyond the financial and geographical reach of many Euro-Canadian settlers. For that reason, many of them continued to rely on alternatives. This was the case for Euro-Canadian women who arrived in western Canada in the late nineteenth century to help establish houses and farms in isolated districts of this so-called Garden of Eden. Lacking organized Western health care, they turned to home remedies passed down by their mothers, to the doctor's books they brought with them, to their neighbours, and – most important – to the local Aboriginal women, who were willing to offer these outsiders their skills in childbirth and plant knowledge.[15] Familiarity, comfort, and gender all played powerful roles in determining the health care preferences of Euro-Canadian women across the Canadian west. Indeed, these women were often more at ease with an experienced healer or midwife than with a male physician, even if that healer or midwife was not white.[16]

Studies conducted outside Canada suggest that Aboriginal women, who lacked formal nursing training but had a great deal of therapeutic experience and knowledge, did a great deal to create and maintain informal networks of nursing care and assistance in colonial settings. In the United States, Susan Smith, in a study of Black lay midwives, found that most black and some white women preferred a midwife to a Euro-Canadian physician, not just for economic reasons but for cultural ones as well.[17] Smith found that midwives were cheaper; would travel to remote places that doctors would not; provided comfort and support to women before, during, and after the delivery; and would look after household chores while caring for new mothers. In addition, class boundaries did not determine the quality of treatment that women received.[18] Midwives' relationships with their patients differed from those of doctors because doctors more often than not arrived after the labour had begun and departed shortly after the child was born.[19] Karen Flint's work on African healers in Natal, South Africa, presents similar conclusions about Aboriginal medical practitioners.[20] Flint found that white South Africans continued to use African healers despite the growing availability of biomedical practitioners.[21] Poor and physically isolated settlers found it easier to secure the curative skills of African healers than to arrange the expensive services of Western medical doctors. The most popular midwives and healers were respected members of the community who knew the family and were not separated by the same barriers of class and gender as male medical professionals.[22]

MEDICINAL PLANTS AND NURSING CARE

There is compelling evidence that white settlers in western Canada relied on Aboriginal women for their knowledge of plant remedies, nursing care, and healing more generally. The first available records from the West that provide evidence that newcomers called on Aboriginal people for medical treatment have been left to us by fur traders. For example, the chief factor (trading post manager) at Fort Pelly, on the northeast elbow of the Assiniboine River, paid a local Aboriginal woman to treat his employees. An entry in the fort's daily log dated February 14, 1863, indicates that an "old native woman was paid six yards of printed cotton for doctoring Thomas Favell."[23] No European women lived at the fort, and the daily log does not state whether the Aboriginal woman lived there or how the chief factor acquired her services. It *does* suggest that Europeans recognized Aboriginal women's medical knowledge and were willing to pay for it. The log entry also demonstrates that Aboriginal women provided more than simply reproductive labour for fur traders.

Another example comes from Charlotte Selina Bompas, the wife of the well-known Anglican missionary William C. Bompas, who was sent to Fort Simpson in the present-day Northwest Territories by the Church Mission Society (CMS) in 1865 and named bishop of Athabasca in 1874.[24] In 1876, while living at Fort Chipewyan (in present-day northern Alberta), Bompas was faced with a difficult situation when she became very ill in the absence of her husband.[25] She was unable to care for herself but was nursed back to health by a Cree woman named Madeline, with whom she had been trading for food.[26] Bompas went so far as to refer to Madeline as her little wife.[27] Historian Myra Rutherdale provides an insightful analysis of the encounter between Bompas and Madeline, noting that while "intimate relations were not part of the dominant colonial discourse, the context of living in the mission field allowed for a challenge to the preconceived notions held by missionaries."[28]

Other stories describe the timely arrival of Aboriginal women and cast them as heroines. This account, from the 1880s, was left to us by an unnamed woman from the Moosomin District in present-day Saskatchewan:[29]

The Indian woman took in the situation at a glance. She pushed aside the terrified mother and picked up the ailing child. By signs she indicated hot water from the kettle on the stove. Into it she put a pinch of herbs from the pouch slung around her waist. She cooled the brew and forced some of it between the blue lips of the infant. Soon the gasping subsided, and sweat broke to cool the fevered skin. The baby relaxed into a peaceful, natural sleep, cradled in the arms of the crooning Indian woman. That mother to her dying day remained grateful.[30]

Dramatic accounts of this sort in many ways mirror the stories told about district nurses who travelled long distances over difficult roads to arrive at the last minute in the middle of the night to save their patients.[31] Many settlers throughout western Canada would recall that there were one or two Aboriginal women in their district who were regarded as both caregivers and doctors and could be called on in case of emergency. These stories have been collected by local historians only decades after the fact.

Another incident was recorded by François Adam during the summer of 1892. Adam's writes that his wife took ill while he and his family were cutting hay at the east end of Crooked Lake, Saskatchewan. He immediately sent one of his farmhands to fetch Father Bellivaire, the local Roman Catholic priest.[32] Father Bellivaire arrived soon after, accompanied by two Aboriginal women and their children. After setting up their tents, the women entered Adam's house. They carried a collection of various twigs and roots, which they proceeded to steep for several hours before giving the mixture to Mrs. Adam, who drank it and immediately felt better.[33] Although Adam might not have known which Aboriginal women in the area were willing to offer their curative skills, he knew that the neighbourhood priest would know. Networks such as these were a common part of life in the Prairie West, and childbirth and illness offer a lens through which to examine these systems.[34]

There is some evidence that in addition to attending to pregnant, ill, or injured newcomers in Canada's north and west, Aboriginal women shared their knowledge of the medicinal properties of local plants. At the least, settlers observed and incorporated their knowledge. Historians have made similar arguments regarding the early period of the fur trade and the important roles that Aboriginal women played at fur trade forts and for the voyageurs. But this recognition has not been extended to the farmers and ranchers who settled the Prairies less then one hundred years later. Such an analysis is warranted. For example, Effie Storer, who settled in the Battleford District in the 1880s, includes this description in an unpublished manuscript: "Down through the ages the squaws have gathered various roots in their season, and buds from different trees and shrubs which they kept or prepared for medicinal use amongst the tribe. And indeed at times helped the early settlers in their need. Many of the elder women proved quite adept at diagnosis and in prescribing the correct herb-tea, the taste of which was long remembered by the patient as in most cases it proved efficacious. Lint from the cotton wood tree and the hairy fuzz of the anemone seed pod were frequently called into requisition."[35]

As late as the 1960s, when he conducted fieldwork among the Sechelt Nation in British Columbia, Lester Peterson found that elders remembered sharing treatments for rheumatism, arthritis, and tuberculosis with members of the non-Aboriginal community.[36] The continued resort to Aboriginal women's therapeutic expertise was a matter of practical necessity and affordability. Aboriginal women provided essential services at times when no one else was available; indeed, in some cases they assisted doctors and even intervened when Western medicine proved inadequate.

Giving Birth in the West

Married women of a certain age were almost certain to require someone's help when it came to giving birth. When Euro-Canadian women learned they were pregnant, they often made plans to be with female relatives or friends close to their due date. But even the best-laid plans went awry. After her marriage in 1864, Susan Allison lived with her husband, John, on his ranch in the Similkameen Valley in present-day BC.[37] Allison recounts giving birth to two of her children during the late 1860s and early 1870s with the help of Aboriginal midwives. On the first occasion, she had intended to travel to Hope to be with her mother for the birth, but she was caught by surprise when the baby was born two months early. John Allison went to the neighbouring ranch and returned with Suzanne, the sister of one of the Aboriginal workers. When Suzanne arrived, she gave Allison whisky to dull the pain.[38] Allison recalls that "Suzanne was good to me in her way – though I thought her rather unfeeling at the time. She thought that I ought to be as strong as an Indian woman but I was not."[39] Allison's second birth, too, was attended by the wife of an Aboriginal man that her husband knew.[40]

Thirty years later a recent immigrant from Ontario, Annie Greer, had a similar experience. During her first winter in Dauphin, Manitoba, in 1893-94, Greer, living in a log-and-sod hut, was by herself when she went

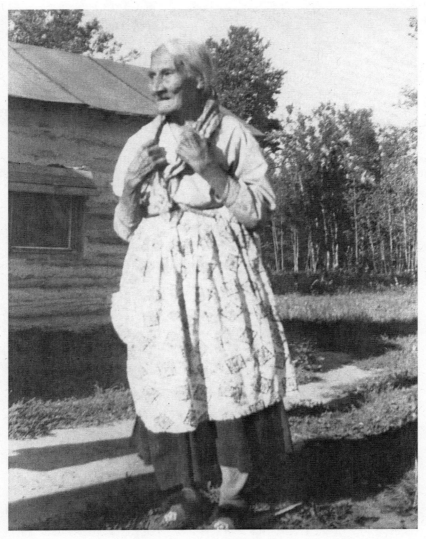

Mrs. Adam Callihou, a Métis woman from Hazelmere, Alberta, who was a midwife for settlers in the area, 1955. | Courtesy Glenbow Archives NA-1271-2

into labour.[41] Greer gave birth to her first child with the assistance of the local midwife, Caroline, who was the wife of the chief at the neighbouring reserve. Caroline came prepared with a satchel full of herbs, roots, bark, and leaves. She saved the mother's life and refused payment for doing so.[42] A decade later Mary Lawrence of northern Alberta made a similar choice when she secured help to deliver her first child. Lawrence preferred an Aboriginal midwife over the alternative at hand – her father-in-law.[43] Statements such as Alison's suggest that although white women were relieved when an Aboriginal woman arrived to attend them, they continued to regard them as a last resort and very different in their manners and thought processes. These practices and beliefs were a way for white women to maintain their separateness from Aboriginal women, notwithstanding the intimate proximity in which childbirth placed them.

Physicians were often unable to reach women in time because few doctors worked in rural districts. Physicians preferred to practise in urban areas, where there was a better chance of making a decent living.[44] Most physicians were not guaranteed a steady income and supplemented their practices with other paid employment.[45] Even DIA doctors could not support themselves on their salaries. Dr. Lafferty, for example, worked as the medical officer for the Blackfoot for more than twenty years. But he also had a practice in Calgary, ran a ranch, was a banker, ran a dry-goods store, and was periodically the mayor of Calgary.[46]

Effie Storer used the obstetrical services of an Aboriginal woman while stationed at Whitefish Lake (in present-day Alberta) with her husband, a NWMP officer. Storer recalled that her daughter, Irene, was born on March 30, 1894. Since the closest doctor lived in Edmonton, she was compelled to rely on the services of an "old medicine woman."[47] The following year, when her husband was transferred to Battleford (in present-day Saskatchewan), her daughter, Muriel, was born prematurely. Once again, an Aboriginal midwife was called in to oversee the labour.[48] It is noteworthy that during an era when the NWMP were actively involved in restricting the physical movements of Aboriginal people through the pass system, Aboriginal women were able to circumvent these restrictions to attend the wives of NWMP officers.

Some physicians realized that they could not be present at all births and made other arrangements. Kay Thompson, an Assiniboine woman, told historian Maureen Lux about Mrs. Walker, an experienced midwife and medicine woman, who had attended many successful births at the reserve. Dr. Isman, the physician from the village of Wolseley, Saskatchewan, had often asked Walker to manage those births he was unable to attend.[49] That some doctors appreciated the expertise of Aboriginal midwives is evident in the reminiscence of a Cree woman about her mother, Harriet Sayese, a midwife who lived near Frog Lake: "Mother although she never received an education, was wonderful help and much was accomplished among our Native people on the reserve. When people were sick mother was called on to help, often being midwife. She even helped Dr. Miller at times, as midwife, in the old hospital he had set up in his home at Elk Point in the early 1920s."[50]

Indeed, throughout the Canadian west, doctors who knew they would be unable to attend all births – especially in isolated locations – came to rely on local midwives. Ellen Smallboy, a Cree woman, born in 1853 near James Bay, remembered that the Indian agent, a doctor, had taught one of the midwives at the reserve techniques that enabled her to be more adept at dealing with difficult obstetrical cases.[51]

Doctors themselves often did not possess the training or experience for complicated obstetrical cases. In their article on childbirth and hospitalization in Vancouver, Veronica Strong-Boag and Kathryn McPherson write that appropriate obstetrical training for doctors remained a problem well into the twentieth century.[52] At Vancouver General Hospital, for instance, interns were given only two months of training on the maternity ward. After that, they had to seek out extra training or practise on their own.[53] The lack of attention paid to obstetrics in medical school was contrary to the realities of general practice, a large part of which involved women and their pregnancies. During the late nineteenth and early twentieth centuries, settlers in Saskatchewan identified childbirth as the most common reason for family members' being bedridden and needing the attention of a doctor.[54] Because so many doctors lacked the necessary training, in remote locations they called on experienced midwives to "assist" them during maternity calls.

In light of doctors' inadequate obstetrical training, it is not surprising that the knowledge of experienced local midwives was an important resource for doctors who worked far from hospitals. For example, Irene Farwell Bradley, a well-known midwife in Newfoundland, was approached by Dr. Gerald Smith, who asked her if she could help him with his maternity cases.[55] In the West midwives often attended maternity cases with doctors.[56] Ethel Jameson, who lived in Melfort, Saskatchewan, noted in 1901 that since the local doctor was relatively young and inexperienced when it came to maternity cases, he was always accompanied by an experienced midwife.[57] In the pioneer questionnaire conducted by the Saskatchewan Archives Board (SAB) in the 1950s, some women stated that they preferred those doctors who worked with midwives.[58] Certain midwives were recognized as experts on childbirth; certain doctors were not.

Some historians have characterized the rise of obstetrics as a medical speciality in the early twentieth century, in tandem with the desire for physicians to control the field, as the catalyst for midwifery's decline in

Canada. Indeed, that particular women's skill set was eventually banned, and only recently has that ban been lifted. Historian Lesley Biggs tells us, however, that the decline of midwifery was uneven across the country.[59] Urban centres such as Toronto and Montreal saw a sharp and early decline in the practice, whereas midwifery continued to be practised in more remote areas that were desperate for any medical attendance. As a result, less populated and rural regions of Canada, including the Prairie West, experienced the decline of midwifery quite differently.

Geography was not the only factor constraining Euro-Canadians' access to physicians and hospitals in Canada. Statistics collected by the Women's Branch of the United Farmers of Manitoba indicated that, prior to 1920, a doctor's visit could cost anywhere from twenty-five to fifty dollars.[60] The SAB questionnaire found that childbirth was not only the most common medical expense for families but also the most costly. A maternity case could cost anywhere from ten to sixty dollars, depending on the distance travelled by the doctor and the length of time he attended the birth.[61] Given the boom-and-bust nature of the West's economy, few farmers could afford to summon a doctor. In addition, many settlers who wanted to use a hospital could not do so because the cost of inpatient care was prohibitive. Not until 1917, under the Municipal Hospitalization Plan, were stays in Alberta hospitals subsidized by the provincial government. For standard ward care, the charge was one to two dollars a day.[62]

Familiarity and comfort also drove the choices that Euro-Canadian women made about their birth attendants. There are several reported cases of women in southern Saskatchewan preferring a skilled midwife to the medical alternatives, even when the latter were available to them. Mrs. White and Mrs. Hubbard said that there were only three doctors in their district: one was very nice but old and deaf; another had been a doctor in the army and had little patience for women; and the third drank too much.[63]

In other cases Aboriginal women were preferred because they had close ties with the community and were widely known to be successful midwives and healers. Female settlers would often remember the important caregiving functions of Aboriginal women in their communities. A Euro-Canadian woman who lived in Saskatchewan's Rocanville District in the late 1880s fondly remembered a Cree woman who had been called whenever there was a birth in the family and who had acted as the district's general nurse.[64] The nearest doctor was at least thirty miles away and charged fifteen dollars for a maternity visit. Another Euro-Canadian woman warmly remembered relying on a "nice old Cree lady, Mrs. Fisher, from across the lake, who acted as both doctor and nurse for the neighbourhood."[65] Mrs. Fisher could not speak English. Even so, because the nearest doctor was at Qu'Appelle, she was called whenever there was a birth. As with physicians, some midwives were in higher demand than others. Ellen Smallboy remembered that some women such as her sister Harriet and her sister-in-law Christina "were more adept than others" and were called more often.[66]

At the turn of the century, another option became available to women of the Prairie West – maternity homes. Those in western Canada differed sharply from those in central Canada during the mid-nineteenth century. The activities of eastern maternity homes were deeply rooted in the social reform movement. In contrast, maternity homes on the Prairies were not run by charities designed to save so-called fallen women. They were private services made available by individual women that mainly provided childbirth expertise. Most of these homes were in rural areas – that is, in communities that were too small to attract doctors or to support a hospital.[67] Many women, however, could not afford the convenience of these homes. Another drawback to maternity homes was that they pulled women away from their families for long periods of time. Winnifred Taylor, for instance, had her first child at a private nursing home in North Battleford and found that she did not like this option because it meant being away from home for over a month (she had left home two weeks early to ensure she arrived on time).[68]

Well into the twentieth century, geography, cost, and preference factored greatly in the medical options open to women. In 1926 in Canada, only 17.8 percent of births took place in a hospital. The vast majority continued to occur in the home.[69] A study of maternal mortality in Canada in the early 1920s found that only 14 percent of the cases included in the survey were attended by doctors. Most often, the doctor was not called until several days after the birth – usually not until it was clear that the patient was dying.[70] Settlers often viewed doctors as a last resort. As a child in Pheasant Forks (located in present-day Saskatchewan) in the 1880s, Edith Mary Stillborne viewed a doctor's call as a prelude to death.[71] In the late nineteenth and early twentieth centuries, Canadian women rarely used hospitals for childbirth. Only single mothers and women without the financial means to support a healthy home birth used hospitals.[72] Ella Mott, who lived in the Qu'Appelle District of Saskatchewan during the 1880s, believed that "only beggars were born in a hospital." Everyone else was born at home.[73] Even for those women who had a home and family support, midwives remained a welcome alternative. As late as the 1930s, many settler women in the West preferred Aboriginal healers and midwives to hospital care.[74]

ABORIGINAL WOMEN'S HEALTH WORK IN ALBERTA

The exchange of healing skills and health knowledge documented in Canada's western and northern regions were also evident in southern Alberta during the late nineteenth century. Aboriginal women provided Euro-Canadians who lived in Alberta with healing services. In 1847 Robert T. Rundle, the first Methodist missionary in Fort Edmonton (having arrived in 1840), fell from his horse and broke his arm while visiting the Blackfoot. Blackfoot healers set Rundle's arm and cared for him.[75] John Maclean, the Methodist missionary at the Blood Reserve, was known to make use of Aboriginal people's medical knowledge. In 1888 his wife, Sara Ann, cut her finger, which became infected.[76] Before he left to travel his circuit, he advised her to see the local Aboriginal healer and commented that the problem would be cleared up in less than a week if she did. Unfortunately for Sara Ann, she did not follow her husband's advice and was forced to have her finger removed at the knuckle. It is not recorded who performed the amputation.[77] Another acknowledgment of Aboriginal healing appears in a diary entry made by Maclean in December 1888, in which he records the presence of a sick cowboy in one of the camps and notes that he is being cared for by a Blackfoot family in their home and attended by an "old medicine woman."[78] Sometimes the local priest or missionary retained the services of Aboriginal women for white settlers – for example, he might bring several Aboriginal women to treat a settler's sick wife.[79]

A final aspect of newcomers' encounters with Aboriginal people was the sharing of local botanical knowledge. As the last chapter describes, the activities of Aboriginal women were much less visible that those of buffalo-hunting warrior men. The work of Aboriginal women, who collected berries and dug up roots, was obscured by the physical landscape of the West. For Euro-Canadian women to see or learn about Aboriginal women's plant remedies, a certain proximity was necessary. Euro-Canadian women would have had to seek out Aboriginal women to acquire this knowledge. Only close contact would have enabled them to learn which plants to use, when to harvest them, and how to administer them.

The case of Marie Rose Smith illustrates that Euro-Canadian women observed or were aware of Aboriginal women's botanical knowledge. Smith was a Métis from Winnipeg who married a white fur trader and settled in Pincher Creek, Alberta. She was familiar with certain treatments the Blackfoot used to cure physical ailments. In an unpublished manuscript she writes that the Blackfoot "scraped the [bark] of the poplar tree, which [was] very bitter, but white and mix[ed] it with a little water to be used as a cathartic [and] for muscular ailment, [the Blackfoot] built sweat houses of willow sticks, covered with buffalo hides."[80] Smith's manuscript, however, contains no specific reference to interactions with Aboriginal women. Similarly, a local history of southern Alberta notes that the Blackfoot used a "ball shaped fungus, similar to a mushroom, which ... when tied over a wound would stop bleeding and was used as an anaesthetic."[81] Settlers who recounted this type of information never indicated *who* they acquired it from. The anonymity of the sources suggests that early settlers made claim to being real pioneers by gaining possession of elements of Aboriginal people's environmental knowledge. Perhaps these silences were meant to imply that, as pioneers, their information came from a vanished and noble race, one quite different from contemporary Aboriginal people as Euro-Canadians viewed them.

There were times when the healing expertise of Aboriginal women was resorted to after Western medicine proved ineffective. Saskatchewan settler Charles Bray remembered a time when his sister-in-law was suffering from dysentery. Her local doctor could find no cure, but a Blackfoot woman steeped a tea of white prairie flowers. Bray's sister drank it and recovered.[82] Clearly, it was not only Aboriginal people who chose their medical treatments based on effectiveness. Given the state of Western medicine in the late nineteenth century, it was not unusual for Euro-Canadian settlers to seek other alternatives when allopathic medicine and Western physicians failed them.

As in other settler regions, many Euro-Canadian women in Canada had no choice but to give birth and raise their children far from familial support. For example, in the Bow River District of southern Alberta there were 3,275 people in 1880-81, of whom 180 were English, 100 were French, and 90 were of "various other origins." The rest were Aboriginal people.[83] The 400 non-Aboriginal people were spread out across ranches and farms at least 160 acres in size. As many scholars have noted, the Dominion Survey, intended to transform and settle western space, in its application ensured a thinly spread out settler population that lived on isolated farms.[84]

One consequence was that Euro-Canadian women relied on Aboriginal women for help during childbirth. Mary Cecil, a Cree midwife, attended

Eliza Boyd, the wife of the well-known Methodist missionary John McDougall, and her sister-in-law Annie McDougall, when they gave birth to their children at the Stoney Reserve. Cecil worked for the McDougalls as a midwife, nurse, and servant for many years.[85] Annie McDougall remembered Mary affectionately and wrote that although she had initially feared her, "she ... soon become very fond of [Mary] because of her kindness and faithfulness. For twenty eight years I had no better servant or friend, and the children loved her as well as any white woman."[86]

The wives of government employees also made use of the obstetrical skills of local Aboriginal women. Like agricultural families, Indian agents and their wives lived in isolated and under-serviced communities. F.C. Cornish, the Indian agent for the Sarcee Reserve from 1887 to 1890, in his unpublished reminiscences recalls that his eldest son was born while he was employed at the Sarcee Reserve. "In those days," he writes, "it was not an easy matter making provision for such an event. The nearest doctor was in Calgary. Nurses were unattainable."[87] Mrs. Cornish had been able to obtain the obstetrical services of the interpreter's wife, a Tsuu T'ina woman, who was well known as a good midwife.[88]

Aboriginal women sometimes provided Euro-Canadian women with advice about birth control and abortion. Historian Eliane Silverman carried out a series of interviews with women who had lived in Alberta at the turn of the century. She found evidence that Aboriginal women shared knowledge with non-Aboriginal people about abortion. One woman revealed what she had heard about how Aboriginal women dealt with birth control: "I guess the priests didn't approve, but the woman figures that's the Indian way, not the white man's way. They sewed a black bag from the bladder of a bear. They'd dry it, then mix it with some liquid, and then they'd lose the baby. There must be some medicine in that. They figure that's okay. It's from the land, they figure it didn't do any harm. Well the priest didn't know about it. Nobody told him about it."[89]

These stories from southern Alberta, in conjunction with evidence from western Canada in general, confirm that obstetrical and healing work created a space in which Aboriginal and Euro-Canadian women came together. It is difficult, though, to determine the frequency and intensity of these encounters. In some sense, Aboriginal women's caregiving work seems to have been a logical extension of the other labouring tasks they performed in southern Alberta. Aboriginal peoples – especially the Nakoda – worked on the farms and ranches of Euro-Canadian settlers in southern Alberta.[90] The letters of Monica Hopkins, an immigrant from

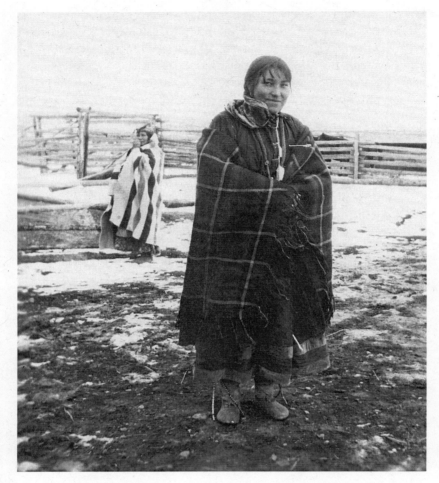

Mrs. John Bearspaw on Basilici Ranch, Kew, Alberta, 1916. | Courtesy Glenbow Archives NA-3917-55

England and a rancher's wife in southern Alberta, reveal that each time the Hopkins hired Peter Bearspaw as a seasonal labourer, he brought his entire family with him – four men and seven children.[91] Hopkins shared her food with the Bearspaw family and even played the gramophone for Peter and his family on a special occasion. Bearspaw's family stayed for several weeks, and Hopkins missed the children when they returned to the Morley reserve.[92]

Aboriginal women performed washing, sewing, cleaning, and other sorts of domestic labour for Euro-Canadian women who lived near

Treaty 7 reserves.[93] Annual departmental reports reveal that Aboriginal men participated in local ranching and seasonal economies.[94] They delivered supplies, hauled coal and wood for the NWMP, and worked as farm and ranch hands for local settlers.[95] Some ranching families in southern Alberta formed enduring economic and social relationships with Aboriginal families. In particular, the Nakoda who worked as seasonal labourers for ranchers tended to form special ties, sanctioned by the band, with particular ranching families. The Rider family was associated with the Bar U, the Bearspaws were associated with the Bedingfelds, and the Dixons were associated with the Gardners.[96] Given these extensive economic and social ties, we should not be surprised that Aboriginal women were willing to offer their help with childbirth and healing.

Despite the importance of Aboriginal women's help, Euro-Canadians were reluctant to acknowledge it. To this day, silence persists regarding the healing and caregiving interventions of Aboriginal women. The McDougall women provide the most obvious example of this historical silence. When they were invited to speak about their experiences, the stories they told did not include the work of Aboriginal women. When Eliza McDougall gave an address at the evening service of the Pincher Creek United Church on June 6, 1935, she described the deprivation experienced by the wives of missionaries: "In the main the men could take care of themselves, but what of women? Without companionship of their own sex, except the squaws, sharing all the hardship and privations of frontier life, bearing their children without medical or nursing aid, these are some of the sacrifices made by the noble generation of women."[97]

Indeed, of the nearly twenty addresses to church audiences that Eliza McDougall and her sister-in-law Annie delivered, none mention the women's close and important relationships with Aboriginal women. Nor does John McDougall's publication mention intimate encounters with Aboriginal women – for example, that his oldest children were of mixed race descent because his first wife, Abigail, was an Ojibwa-Cree woman. In an interview with journalist Elizabeth Bailey Price in the late 1920s, Annie McDougall revealed that Mary Cecil had been very important in ensuring the well-being of the McDougall women. Was this disclosure a result of the reporter's questions or of Annie's desire to set the record straight? The latter is most likely.

Departmental correspondence likewise fails to note that Indian agent Cornish's wife relied on an Aboriginal midwife. Rather, the Aboriginal midwife emerges in undated reminiscences penned by Cornish and stored at the Glenbow Archives years later.[98] Similarly, John Maclean's advice to his wife that she consult an Aboriginal healer is documented in personal correspondence, while his speeches and published texts represent Aboriginal healing practices as "medical folk-lore" and superstitious beliefs that rely on harmless objects to affect cures.[99] Maclean's works, like other missionary texts from the time, portray Aboriginal traditions of therapeutic knowledge as ineffective and hazardous.[100]

Euro-Canadian women and their husbands eulogized white women's roles as harbingers of civilization and lamented their lack of white female companionship and want of proper medical care. Historian Jennifer Brown points to a comparable silence in the published texts of Egerton Ryerson Young, who did not acknowledge the influential role the Cree nanny, Little Mary, played in his son's life.[101] Andrea Smith calls the invisibility of Aboriginal women in the colonial imagination a present absence.[102] It is not surprising, then, that evidence of Aboriginal women's midwifery and healing sits uneasily among broader colonial narratives about the process of settlement and nation building. Settler women only begrudgingly acknowledged their debt to the Aboriginal women who helped them.

Acknowledging the labour of Aboriginal women might have been especially awkward given the growing efforts to restrain Aboriginal women in their own communities and homes. As an employee of the DIA, Cornish was responsible for stamping out Aboriginal cultural activities, and Mrs. Cornish was expected to teach Aboriginal women European values and domestic skills.[103] They might have felt conflicted about relying on Aboriginal women's healing skills, and it is possible that their employer did not look favourably on such activities. Prior to 1884 the Indian Act had dealt mainly with issues of property acquisition and disposal, Indian government, and education.[104] But an 1885 amendment banned the potlatch and all giveaway ceremonies. The Act was amended further in 1895 (section 114) to prohibit the okan (Sun Dance) and similar ceremonies. These amendments provided agents with the necessary legal tools to suppress Aboriginal medicine and culture. Moreover, the curative and domestic practices of Aboriginal women were seen by the DIA as integral to cultural persistence. When Aboriginal women continued to draw upon these traditions, they were increasingly regarded as the root of the communities' lack of progress. Women thus became particular targets for change. Recognizing that Aboriginal women had important domestic skills would have challenged the ideological underpinnings of the colonial project.[105]

Negative images of Aboriginal women led many westerners to regard their very presence in cities and towns as a social and moral concern.[106] The stereotype of Aboriginal women as shameless prostitutes was especially powerful.[107] After 1892 the Criminal Code and the Indian Act made it easier to convict Aboriginal women for prostitution. Local incidents such as the one in 1884, when Aboriginal women were denied access to a ball held at Fort Macleod's NWMP barracks, reflected popular mechanisms for constraining Aboriginal women's movements. In 1885 a Native woman in Battleford (in present-day Saskatchewan) had her hair chopped off as punishment for being in town without a pass.[108] In Calgary town residents were cautioned against hiring Aboriginal women or buying anything from them.[109]

That missionaries and Indian agents and their families welcomed Aboriginal women into their homes in these circumstances suggests a tremendous need for health care among Euro-Canadians. It also highlights the uneven effects of colonial power. It is possible that interactions between Aboriginal and Euro-Canadian women had declined by the end of the nineteenth century. In a study of childbirth on the Canadian prairies, Nanci Langford examines the diaries and letters of seventy-eight female homesteaders in Saskatchewan and Alberta. Of those seventy-eight women, only two called on Aboriginal women as birth attendants. Note, however, that most of the documents examined by Langford relate to the decades after 1900, when Euro-Canadian settlements were neither as small nor as isolated as in previous decades.[110]

Conclusion

It is clear that some Euro-Canadians were reluctant to record their reliance on southern Alberta's Aboriginal women. Generally, though, the evidence suggests that between 1870 and 1900 Aboriginal and Euro-Canadian women often encountered one another in settlers' homes as a consequence of the gender-specific demands that female newcomers faced when it came to domestic healing and nursing care. Indeed, intimate interactions with Aboriginal women are proof of the difficulties that Euro-Canadian women faced as they helped their men settle the West. Popular discourse might have privileged white identity, but the harsh realities of life in the early West made transparent the different ways that newcomer women experienced settlement. At the same time, gender shaped both the work that Aboriginal people performed and the spaces they occupied. The kinds of work they performed allowed them access to the private and female-centred spaces of Euro-Canadian settlers. Moreover, in light of the silences that persist about such encounters, when examples of health-based interactions do appear – perhaps as a result of the slipping point between formal and informal writing – they suggest that these contacts were more pervasive than the evidence implies.

Will we ever know how Aboriginal women such as Mary Cecil felt about being made invisible? There are no records that indicate how Aboriginal women reacted to this lack of acknowledgment. Available materials only allow the work to become visible. They do not provide insight into Aboriginal women's thoughts and feelings. The growth of missionary medical work and Western medical institutions after the 1890s further obscured the curative work of Aboriginal women and challenged the place of informal care networks in the West. Colonialism marginalized and denigrated Aboriginal culture in part by obscuring the importance of Aboriginal women and their work.

4
Converging Therapeutic Systems

Encounters between Aboriginal and Non-Aboriginal Women, 1870s-90s

At the time that Aboriginal women were making their therapeutic expertise available to newcomers, the social, political, and economic landscape of the West – southern Alberta in particular – was undergoing dramatic changes. During the 1870s and 1880s, the numbered treaties were negotiated, reserves were created, and the Department of Indian Affairs (DIA) – and its bureaucracy – became a force in the West. These decades also saw the founding of medical institutions in white settlements and the growing presence of Western health personnel. Aboriginal people made use of white communities' medical facilities as well as the healing and nursing care provided by female missionaries and missionaries' wives on reserves. The presence of church and state medical services on reserves and the proximity of physicians and medical facilities in nearby Euro-Canadian communities provided Aboriginal people with a broader range of health care choices. At the same time, however, these developments led to new restrictions on Aboriginal people's access to non-Aboriginal institutions, including medical ones.

Euro-Canadians had begun to build hospitals in southern Alberta by the 1870s. The first of these were either founded to care for miners and railway workers or infirmaries for local North West Mounted Police (NWMP) detachments. Over time these facilities extended their services to the surrounding communities. Around the same time, the DIA began to develop a policy (or lack thereof) regarding medical services for Aboriginal people. At first, Euro-Canadian women participated in the informal system of healing and nursing care. By the late 1890s, female missionaries were making medical and nursing care available to Aboriginal people at the mission house and in Aboriginal people's homes and camps. The mission station and the healing and nursing work of female missionaries and missionaries' wives came to be important to Aboriginal communities during a time of diminishing resources. At the same time, the informal, unstructured health work of Aboriginal and non-Aboriginal women fostered moments of contact centred on health care in western Canada. The health care work of Euro-Canadian women remained closely linked to their Christian mission and their efforts to transform Aboriginal society. This informal curative and nursing labour by Euro-Canadians was an important precursor to later health care regimes operated by the colonial state.

Healing Encounters on the Reserve

Unlike the federal government, missionary organizations did not hesitate to involve themselves in the medical care and physical well-being of Aboriginal people. From the time they arrived on the northwestern Plains, male missionaries and their wives participated in the informal network of nursing care and medical aid that stretched across the Prairies. At the same time, Aboriginal women provided missionaries' wives with midwifery and nursing care, and male missionaries turned to Aboriginal healers when they were injured. After the 1880s Euro-Canadian women began to arrive on reserves, where they offered basic first aid, medicine, and caregiving to Aboriginal people at the mission house. At first this labour was an extension of the informal network of mutual aid between Aboriginal people and newcomers. However, the medical and nursing care that the missionaries made available did not come without strings: it was closely linked to missionaries' efforts to Christianize and civilize Aboriginal people. Mission medicine in Canada, as in other European colonies, embraced the perspective that disease and ill health could only be eradicated by embracing Christian morality, a European version of family life, and appropriate gender roles.[1] In return for medical assistance and nursing care, missionaries' wives and female missionaries expected Aboriginal children to attend the church's day schools. They also expected Aboriginal women to be present at the informal prayer and educational gatherings held at the mission house. The informal health care made available by female missionaries can therefore be seen as the forerunner of institutional public health regimes established after the 1890s.

Missionary societies in Britain and Canada began to send men to work in the Canadian northwest as early as the 1840s. The first missionaries to reach Fort Edmonton were Robert Rundle, a Methodist, in 1840, and Jean-Baptiste Thibault, a Catholic priest, in 1842.[2] Mission work during this early period was daunting, given the mobile nature of Plains people. Missionaries were required to travel with Aboriginal groups, learn their languages, and live in isolated areas.[3] The masculine nature of early mission work often discouraged Euro-Canadian women, married or otherwise, from joining their male counterparts. The arrival of Euro-Canadian women in the late 1870s and early 1880s transformed the place of healing and nursing care within the missionary enterprise. Once Euro-Canadian women arrived on the scene, Western medicine became more important to missionary work, and the growing number of white women in the field reflected this development. By 1900, one-third of the Protestant missionaries in the Canadian west were women.[4] And the medical and nursing aspects of mission work were heavily dominated by women.

The latter half of the nineteenth century witnessed the emergence of a new field of mission activity – women's work for women. This activity was grounded in good works and so-called social housekeeping. The perception was that this type of work was instinctive to European women, who were caregivers by nature.[5] Conversions were the province of male missionaries; women had to prove their usefulness in other ways. To do so, they focused on roles regarded as essentially female, such as nursing and education. Drawing from universal ideas of maternalism, European women constructed responsibilities for themselves in the mission field that over time became irreplaceable. They came to be seen as the best candidates for the job not only because they were believed to be natural caregivers but also because mission societies hoped that woman-to-woman connections would give missionaries the opportunity to enter sites of activity previously forbidden to men. Over time it became clear that the churches were failing to convert and assimilate Aboriginal peoples. On its own, proselytizing was not enough to attract Aboriginal people to the fold. So mission societies placed more importance on alternative approaches. In this regard, the healing and caregiving work of European women became essential to the churches' work in western Canada. In communities that were in desperate need of social and economic relief, the services offered by European women became essential.

At first glance, this growing field of activity seemed designed to address the medical and health needs of Aboriginal populations in crisis. In practice, however, the primary objective of health care delivery remained the dissemination of Christianity and Euro-Canadian culture.[6] Indeed, white women's health work offered the perfect opportunity to introduce Aboriginal people to middle-class Euro-Canadian understandings of appropriate forms of domestic and personal hygiene and child care. As a result, Christianity and civilization became directly linked to the practice and use of Western medicine in the mission field. Moreover, Aboriginal women who chose to avail themselves of Western medicine were in the eyes of missionaries symbolically accepting all of the cultural baggage that Western medicine represented. In this manner women's health work became equally important, if not more important, in the acquisition of Aboriginal souls and the assimilation of Aboriginal peoples.

Missions were established at the five reserves in southern Alberta by the end of the 1880s. Some reserves had multiple Christian denominations competing for Aboriginal souls. As historian John Webster Grant writes, the treaties "constituted a charter of missionary advance" in that they allowed missionary organizations greater influence over a population that was increasingly segregated and immobilized.[7] Ministering to Aboriginal people confined to reserves, especially after 1885, required a different type of missionary. For Protestants this new ideal missionary was expected to fill a number of roles and perform multiple functions: he should be married to serve as an example of Christian domesticity; he should be a steady pastor to his congregation; he should be able to attract the interest of women's organizations, whose fundraising and spiritual support was vital to missions during this period; he should be able to direct a female labour force, which did most of the teaching and nursing; and he should be able to work closely with government agents and farm instructors as a competent administrator. For Roman Catholic missionaries the situation was slightly different: women's work remained central, but the commitment to providing an example of married Christian domesticity was obviously less relevant. Women religious stood as examples of Christian womanhood, and their work in hospitals, school infirmaries, and dispensaries served as examples of cleanliness and domesticity. Priests might have administered the mission broadly, but the day-to-day management of individual institutions was left almost entirely to Catholic sisterhoods. After 1880 both Protestants and Catholics were required to be able administrators.

The Methodist Church

The Methodists were very active in western Canada during the mid- and late nineteenth century. In 1873 a permanent mission was built by John

McDougall and his wife, Eliza Boyd McDougall, among the Nakoda at Morleyville. John McDougall had been an active participant in the Treaty 7 negotiations, during which he served as a translator for the treaty commissioners. McDougall, a proponent of settlement, urged southern Alberta's Aboriginal peoples to accept the treaty and adopt an agricultural lifestyle. His role in the treaty-making process remains extremely controversial because he exemplified those missionaries whose interests went beyond ministering to their flocks.[8] In 1875 he established the McDougall Residential School (also referred to as the McDougall Orphanage). The Methodist Women's Missionary Society (WMS) supported the mission and school at Morley. The WMS paid the salaries of a field matron, a nurse, and female teachers. In 1906 the same organization helped found the reserve's short-lived Methodist hospital, which was run by one female nurse until it closed. Without the WMS this mission would not have survived as long as it did.

In 1880 the Reverend John Maclean founded a Methodist mission among the Kainai. Maclean was accompanied by his wife, Sara Ann Barker, who spent a great deal of her time travelling with her husband to the camps. During these visits Barker offered first aid and domestic instruction to Kainai women. Barker regularly used her home as a place to nurse sick people. The Macleans left the Blood Reserve in 1889, and the Methodist mission did not long survive their departure.[9]

The Roman Catholic Church

The Missionary Oblates of Mary Immaculate were responsible for most of the Roman Catholic missionary work in Alberta. With the capable assistance of the Sisters of Charity of Montreal (a.k.a. the Grey Nuns), who arrived at Lac Sainte-Anne on September 25, 1859, the Oblates ran residential schools and helped build reserve hospitals throughout Alberta.[10] The Grey Nuns possessed a great deal of experience running hospitals and nursing the sick. Besides doing hospital work, they helped the Oblates run residential schools.[11] When the Oblates established St. Joseph's Industrial School (commonly known as Dunbow) east of High River in 1884, the Grey Nuns joined them. At Dunbow the sisters served as teachers, housekeepers, child care providers, and nurses in the school's small infirmary. The school closed in 1924. The sisters assumed similar responsibilities at the Sacred Heart Residential School, which was opened in 1897 at the Peigan Reserve. At the Blood Reserve, the sisters opened and ran a small hospital in 1894.

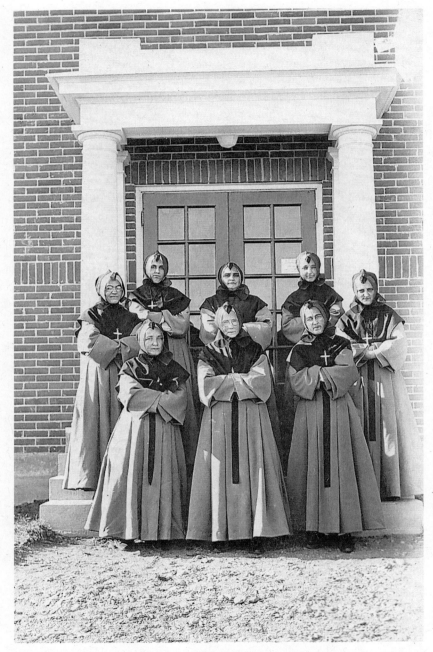

Grey Nuns standing on the steps of the Blood Hospital, 1920s. | Courtesy Grey Nuns Archives, Montreal

The Anglican Church

The final denomination to undertake mission work among the northwestern Plains people of southern Alberta was the Anglican Church. The Anglican Church was relatively slow to harness the work of women in the mission field. Not until the 1880s did the Domestic and Foreign Mission Societies begin to actively recruit single Euro-Canadian women, building on the idea of women's work for women. Women secured their importance in the mission field through teaching and by working as matrons, housekeepers, and nurses. The first Anglican organization to send a female missionary to the North-West Territories was Toronto's Church Women's Mission Aid Society, the first female-led institution within the Anglican Church. In 1879 the society's Toronto group sent Kate Brown to work as a teacher at the Peigan Reserve and later among the Blackfoot. In April 1887 that group merged with the newly formed National Women's Auxiliary.[12] Over the next twenty years, women's auxiliaries sprang up in cities and towns all over Canada. Individual auxiliaries adopted and almost entirely supported specific missions. The fundraising efforts of these groups were instrumental in supporting missionary work in western Canada.

The Anglicans were especially eager to establish schools among the Treaty 7 nations. During the nineteenth century, they founded a mission at every reserve in southern Alberta except for the Stoney Reserve. The schools usually included a school infirmary or a small cottage hospital, run by female mission workers. The Church Mission Society (CMS) sent Archdeacon J.W. Tims to work among the Siksika in 1883. The Old Sun Residential School was opened shortly after his arrival. Tims also wanted to build a hospital at the Blackfoot Reserve. To that end he approached the Toronto Women's Auxiliary, which agreed to pay for furnishings and a nurse's salary. That group supported this hospital until it was formerly taken over by the DIA in 1923. Tims did not stay to see the fruits of his labours. He was forced to depart the Blackfoot Reserve abruptly in 1895 after the death of one of his pupils. The community blamed Tims for the child's death because he had not called the doctor or notified the student's parents. The child died without seeing either her parents or a doctor.[13] A great deal of animosity was expressed by the Siksika. Tims feared for his life and was granted permission by the CMS to relocate to the Sarcee Reserve, where he remained for the next thirty-five years.

Canon H.W. Gibbon Stocken and his wife, Catherine, began the mission among the Tsuu T'ina in May 1888.[14] The Sarcee Residential School was erected in 1890. Despite his best efforts, Stocken was never able to raise enough funds to build a hospital. Instead, during emergencies he often used the mission house as a makeshift infirmary, where his wife would nurse patients. Stocken reluctantly exchanged missions with Tims in 1895. After replacing Stocken, Tims immediately hired a graduate nurse to work at the residential school, perhaps because of his recent experiences among the Siksika. The history of the Sarcee Residential School was not a happy one. It was closed, and then reopened as a sanatorium in 1921 by Dr. Thomas Murray, the new Indian agent and physician, because every single student had been infected with tuberculosis.[15]

The Anglican missionary Samuel Trivett began work at the Blood Reserve in 1880. He opened several day schools with the assistance of Kate Brown. Like the Anglican mission to the Piikani, the mission to the Kainai was never able to acquire the consistent patronage of the women's auxiliaries. As a result, the Blood mission was unable to build St. Paul's Residential School until 1908. Even maintaining trained personnel in the school infirmary was impossible. The Anglicans considered a hospital on this reserve especially important because of the presence of a Roman Catholic institution in the community. A great deal of sectarian conflict persisted between these two groups throughout this period.

The Work of Missionary Women

Although very few personal letters and diaries exist that recount the work and experiences of female missionaries in western Canada, Protestant publications do include letters from their workers in the field. The *Letter Leaflet*, a magazine founded by the Women's Auxiliary of the Anglican Church to publicize its philanthropic work, and the two organs of the Methodist Church, the *Christian Guardian* and the *Missionary Outlook*, published some of the few first-person accounts available that outline the personal experiences of missionary women in western Canada. The letters were meant to keep congregations informed about the churches' mission activities and to encourage readers to provide financial support. As a result the letters often say more about what missionaries believed congregations and potential funding organizations wanted to hear. Accurate representations of Aboriginal people's reactions to and need for missionaries' medical services are generally missing. Even so, these letters when read alongside other materials help us map out the labour of white women at mission stations and hospitals.

The letters of single female missionaries, missionaries' wives, and male missionaries are rife with accounts of the informal healing work performed by Euro-Canadian women at mission stations. According to these published reports, reserve residents – especially before the 1890s – resorted to the mission stations and the women who worked in them for medical and nursing care. John Maclean, a prolific writer who often wrote about the quiet heroism of female missionaries, noted that his wife never turned away any Aboriginal person who came to the mission house seeking first aid.[16] Kate Brown assisted the Reverend H.T. Bourne at the day school at the Peigan Reserve in 1891 and later recounted that Aboriginal people constantly came to the mission house to have her wash and dress their sores.[17] In an 1899 contribution to the *Letter Leaflet,* she expresses her frustration at not being able to do more for her patients: "Many old women suffer from rheumatism, and I often wish for flannel to give them. Another of my patients is a little boy with one hip so terribly diseased that he can only get about on his hands and one foot."[18] Mrs. Bourne, the wife of the missionary at the Peigan Reserve, offers equally heart-rending tales of her work at the mission in 1890: "The bad sores are the most cases we have to treat, [one baby] who is very ill with dreadful sores cries whenever hot poultices are placed on her neck."[19]

Missionary women often opened up the mission house to Aboriginal people, especially children, to provide bedside care. In 1896 Mrs. Stocken and the single female missionary posted with the Siksika were kept busy night and day for three months caring for people in the mission house who suffered from rheumatism, ophthalmia (inflammation of the eye), and a sprained ankle.[20] Ophthalmia was most common in newborns and was directly related to living conditions and inadequate medical treatment. At the Peigan Reserve, visitors to the mission who needed constant nursing care slept in a shanty near the station, where the missionary's wife could attend them and ensure that they received extra food and milk.[21] Kate Brown took into her home the small child of a woman who was too sick to care for the baby herself.[22]

Visiting a mission station may have become one strategy adopted by Aboriginal people seeking Western medical aid and nursing care. The mission house was an agreeable alternative to the institutional settings of the cottage hospital and the school infirmary. At the Blood Reserve, even after the Anglican-run hospital was opened, a dying woman was kept at the mission house, where she was looked after by Mrs. Stocken because "hopeless cases [could not] be admitted to the hospital, the Indians being so superstitious."²³ The care provided by missionary women in their own homes was similar in some respects to the ministering that Aboriginal women were performing in the homes of white women in southern Alberta.

Euro-Canadian women offered to teach Aboriginal women a range of Western domestic skills. Some skills were more useful than others and helped Aboriginal women adapt to changing economic and social circumstances. The collapse of the buffalo hunt required women to look for alternative sources of clothing. Crafts such as sewing and knitting were easily incorporated into already existing female domestic roles and enabled Aboriginal women to make money by selling crafts to non-Aboriginal people.²⁴

Single female missionaries, missionaries' wives, and field matrons sought to teach Aboriginal women how to sew and knit because they regarded such skills as appropriate and productive. Knitting and sewing were intended to replace Aboriginal women's other clothes-making activities, especially those that involved the dressing of hides and the creation of Aboriginal forms of dress. An Indian agent criticized Kainai women in a letter to the DIA, contending that the women were spending most of their time in unproductive pursuits such as tanning hides and making moccasins.²⁵ He believed that this preoccupation only exacerbated Aboriginal women's failure to improve their houses. In other words, Aboriginal women were expected to make clothing for their families, but only if that clothing conformed to European norms.

Notwithstanding the complaints of Indian agents, Aboriginal women were eager to adopt these new skills.²⁶ While teaching at the Blackfoot Reserve in 1888, Kate Brown wrote that she was kept busy teaching Aboriginal women how to sew.²⁷ Brown taught five sewing classes a week at the mission house and often supervised children's sewing during the day.²⁸ Her services were in such high demand that she also held weekly sewing and knitting classes at Big Plume's camp.²⁹ After Brown moved from the Blackfoot to the Peigan Reserve, she continued to hold knitting classes.³⁰ In 1904 Mrs. Stocken began teaching three knitting classes a week at the Blackfoot Reserve. She soon found that knitting was so popular that women were coming daily to learn how to turn a heel or make mittens.³¹ Mrs. Stocken went so far as to make arrangements with a storekeeper in Gleichen to sell the products of Siksika women's labour.³²

New skills such as sewing and knitting coincided with diminishing local animal resources such as the bison and thus served as timely additions to Aboriginal women's expertise.³³ A similar argument is made by John

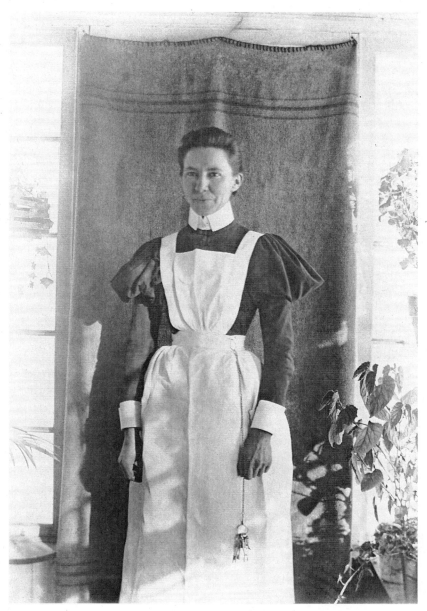

Mrs. Catherine Stocken, Anglican missionary at the Blackfoot Reserve, 1890s. | Courtesy Glenbow Archives NA-1020-9

Lutz, who has examined shifting gender roles over a century of contact in Lekwammen society on the West Coast.[34] Lutz found that changing access to resources prompted Lekwammen women to expand their sewing and knitting activities by adapting their existing knowledge of spinning wool and weaving decorative blankets to the preparation of knitted woollen items.[35] Lekwammen women learned the new skill from immigrants. Historian Sarah Carter likewise notes in her work that Aboriginal women eagerly adopted a wide range of new skills such as milking, butter and bread making, crocheting, knitting, and using sheep's wool to make cloth.[36] It is quite likely that Aboriginal and Euro-Canadian women viewed the adoption of sewing and knitting in highly dissimilar ways. On the one hand, Euro-Canadian women perceived the acceptance of such skills as tangible evidence of change. Aboriginal women most likely saw very little difference between past productive activities and these new ones.

These kinds of interactions show that contact between Aboriginal peoples and Europeans did not end with the decline of the fur trade or the arrival of white women. Instead, the presence of white women marked the onset of encounters among women premised on certain shared female experiences such as reproductive concerns. In situations in which Aboriginal women visited settler and missionary women to provide or receive health services and valuable economic skills, Euro-Canadian homes briefly became places where women encountered one another across the divides of culture and race. In this domestic space, the power relations of colonialism did not disappear; rather, they took a particularly gendered form centred on women's shared domestic responsibilities. Aboriginal women were expected to learn from Euro-Canadian women, not vice versa. When settlers recorded Aboriginal plant knowledge, the inconsistencies of colonialism were exposed.

Aboriginal people are documented as providing Euro-Canadians with instruction about which plants might prove helpful or harmful.[37] Mrs. Reid from Battleford, Saskatchewan, wrote that it was fortunate that there were Aboriginal women who "possessed remarkable knowledge of the simples to be found in the various parts of the West."[38] Likewise, Mrs. Longmore, the wife of Johnny Saskatchewan, was remembered as an Aboriginal woman who "knew all the places where she could gather the leaves, the berries, the barks, and the roots which formed her material medica, and to her knowledge of their efficacy, and skill in their use, many a woman in those days attributed her safe return from the valley of the shadow."[39]

These encounters were less likely to take place in the homes of Aboriginal women. Missionaries' wives did visit Treaty 7 camps to inspect Aboriginal homes, but they justified the visits in terms of evangelical work and domestic instruction. Sara Ann Maclean, the wife of Methodist missionary John Maclean, often accompanied her husband on his visits to the camp to provide Aboriginal women with lessons in domestic economy.[40] Eliza Boyd McDougall, the wife of Methodist missionary John McDougall at the Stoney reserve, wrote about her efforts to teach Aboriginal women who lived nearby how to be good housekeepers.[41] In October 1904 the Methodist missionary Miss Buehler wrote to the WMS that she had made more than fifty home visits to clean and pray with Nakoda residents.[42] The DIA likewise hired a small number of local farm women to visit the homes of Aboriginal women and teach domestic skills.

Mission organizations and the DIA envisioned the work of these women in the homes of Aboriginal people as attempts to transform the domestic space of Aboriginal people and, it followed, the foundations of Aboriginal society. Historian Adele Perry's research shows how "housing became a significant site of conflict in the colonial encounter, a vehicle through which the reorganization of Aboriginal society was imagined, attempted, resisted, and ultimately refashioned."[43] This is not to say that women did not resist the intrusions of Euro-Canadian women into their homes. Margaret Laing, a Methodist mission worker to the Nakoda, remarked that when she tried to instruct Nakoda women about the appropriate way to keep their homes, she was asked not to talk anymore "although the five women who were sitting around could talk all they liked."[44]

The records are not entirely clear about the kinds of work that missionary wives or farm women did when they visited the homes of Treaty 7 people. Hayter Reed, the assistant Indian commissioner from 1883 to 1888, Indian commissioner from 1888-93, and the deputy superintendent general of Indian affairs from 1893 to 1897, did not believe that the work of farm women was having an ameliorative effect on Aboriginal women.[45] In a report to the DIA in 1892, he recommended discontinuing the services of certain farm women because they had failed to carry out inspections to ensure that houses were kept in a clean and orderly manner.[46] What these women actually did is not specified, but it would seem that the contact occurring in Aboriginal women's homes differed significantly from what took place in white women's homes. White women did not spend long periods of time in the tents, teepees, or houses of Aboriginal women: these encounters were brief and solely about domestic instruction.

Relations between European-Canadian and Aboriginal women were also structured differently at the mission schools, although health care remained an important part of white women's work, partly because of the poor conditions that persisted in church-run schools. All mission-run schools offered medical and nursing care to students, often to prevent students from going home, and that aid was provided in the early years by missionary women with no formal nursing training who ran makeshift school infirmaries. At the Stoney Reserve, Miss Barker served as the matron of the McDougall Residential School, which was opened in 1875 by Reverend John McDougall. There, on top of her regular duties, she looked after the children when they became ill. In 1885, when a six-year-old boy died in her care, she had her first experience preparing a body for burial.[47] Only John McDougall's considerable influence in the community kept the remaining children in the school.

Teachers and matrons were often unprepared for the conditions they encountered in mission schools. The schools were often unable to provide their students with proper food and sufficient warm clothing. The letters of female missionaries contain many references to harsh conditions. In letters written in 1895, Kate Brown notes that her teaching work at Peigan Residential School was repeatedly interrupted by nursing duties because the students were often sick with colds and coughs. Brown writes that the school's staff dreaded the appearance of these illnesses. Brown's time was further occupied washing and bandaging the sores of children suffering from scrofula.[48] Half the Piikani children at the mission school were afflicted with that disease, and the missionary's wife, Mrs. Bourne, was kept busy helping Brown tend to the resulting sores. This condition was so rampant that the Women's Auxiliary was forced to hire Mrs. Stuart, a trained nurse, for the winter to help Bourne and Brown.[49] Separated from their families and culture, the children were forced to rely entirely on the Western medical model.

There is no evidence that Aboriginal children were able to turn to Aboriginal therapeutic practices when Western medicine failed them – which it often did. The growth of Western medical services on reserves ensured that medical pluralism could not be practised. Indeed, as historian Mary-Ellen Kelm has aptly observed, the efforts of missionaries and DIA officers to stamp out Aboriginal medicine ensured that the two systems remained distinct.[50] Boundaries of culture and race were rarely if ever transgressed in residential schools, where the full weight of the colonial state was applied to the bodies of Aboriginal children.

Anglican missionaries at the Peigan Reserve constantly negotiated with the Women's Auxiliary to establish a permanent hospital, but it was never built because of lack of secure funding. And the conditions at the Peigan Reserve were not unique. At the Blood Reserve, Mrs. Hardyman, who was the teacher at the small Bull Horn School and the wife of the lay missionary, spent a great deal of her time administering medicine to sick children.[51] Most of the nursing work at the Blood Reserve was eventually taken over by the Grey Nuns, who established and ran a cottage hospital at the reserve in the mid-1890s.

By the close of the century, there was a recognized need for improved health care for the students and the community. Yet, from the missionaries' perspective, nursing work could not be divorced from the larger religious project. As a result some missionaries hesitated to hire trained nurses even after they became available. For instance, when the Anglican residential school at the Sarcee Reserve obtained the appointment of Miss Bella Rutherford, a graduate nurse, in 1897, Rev. Tims, the principal of the school, expressed some reservations regarding her ability to fill the position. Tims was not concerned about Rutherford's nursing qualifications. He did, however, have questions about her practical training in certain domestic tasks such as cooking and housekeeping.[52] In a letter to the secretary of the Christian Missionary Society, he writes:

> I think that the nurse ought to be able to know how to cook for invalids. I should like to know if Miss Rutherford is able to do this. It is not likely that any of the children will always be sick and when there are not patients we would like the nurse to employ her time at needlework and assist in helping the children's clothing repair or making new. There will be ample opportunity for Miss Rutherford to do active mission work amongst both boys and girls. We shall only be too glad to get another earnest Christian engaged in our work here.[53]

Expectations such as Tims's were not unusual. During the nineteenth century, nursing was an occupation performed by a diverse group of women, many of whom included domestic work as part of their repertoire.[54] Tims was happy to have a skilled nurse, but he was also determined to ensure that religious and domestic tasks carried equal weight. When mission societies and their workers had to choose between religion and appropriate health care for Treaty 7 people, religion always came first.

Western Medicine in Southern Alberta before 1890

During the 1870s and 1880s, Western medical services began to develop in southern Alberta. Railway and mining companies erected makeshift hospitals to provide their employees with medical care. Missionary societies and the DIA then built cottage hospitals on Treaty 7 reserves. Aboriginal people often sought out these institutions and their medical personnel.

During the nineteenth century, few settlers had easy or regular access to a physician, a nurse, or a hospital. The first Euro-Canadian women to provide nursing care in Alberta were the Grey Nuns, stationed north of Fort Edmonton at missions in St. Albert and Lac Sainte-Anne. The first hospital in southern Alberta was a small infirmary established at Fort Macleod in 1874 and run by the NWMP.[55] The infirmary was intended to serve NWMP employees, but its reach later expanded to include local settlers and Aboriginal peoples. The infirmary was at first run by the NWMP surgeon and a few male orderlies. But by 1896 local demand for the hospital had grown, and female graduate nurses had taken over the hospital's day-to-day operations.[56]

Hospitals were built in southern Alberta in the 1880s to serve miners and railway workers. In Medicine Hat in 1883, the Canadian Pacific Railway (CPR) built and ran a small infirmary. A makeshift hospital (Coalbanks Mine Hospital) was built in Lethbridge in 1886 and was maintained by the Alberta Railway and Coal Company. The CPR opened a hospital in Banff in 1888 for its employees.[57] Companies built these institutions for their workers. As local populations increased, however, they extended hospital services to settlers.[58] Nursing historian Pauline Paul credits the strong resource-extraction sector for the emergence of a hospital system and the relatively early presence of trained physicians in southern Alberta, compared with the northern portion of the province.[59]

Municipalities took over the operations of some company hospitals in the 1890s. The City of Lethbridge replaced the Coalbanks Hospital with a municipal hospital in 1891. Medicine Hat General Hospital was incorporated by the municipality in 1888 and renovated in 1890.[60] Other municipalities built their own hospitals. Calgary General opened in November 1890 and, the following year, the city founded Holy Cross Hospital.[61] Elizabeth Hoade, a graduate nurse educated in Winnipeg, supervised Calgary General with the help of her husband, who served as night nurse and general caretaker. Holy Cross was run by four nuns from the Sisters of Charity.[62] Women's labour was instrumental in establishing and maintaining the health care facilities that sprang up throughout southern Alberta. They ran the wards, assisted the doctors, administered treatments, provided bedside assistance, and monitored patients' progress.

State Health Care Services

At the same time that hospitals and medical professionals were being established in southern Alberta, the federal government was developing a bureaucracy to manage Aboriginal peoples and their communities. In the 1870s the federal government began intensive efforts to impose European values and institutions on Aboriginal societies.[63] Ottawa was clearly interested in issues of land; it showed much less concern about Aboriginal health. Unlike the churches and mission societies, the DIA showed little interest in the physical well-being of Aboriginal people. Indeed, there are many parallels in western Canada between the federal government's health care programs and its relief programs. In the nineteenth century, when it came to Aboriginal people, the federal state did not view welfare relief as its responsibility. The government feared that so-called state charity would erode Aboriginal peoples' independence.[64] Ottawa regarded medical care as a form of charity and was determined that only the neediest of Aboriginal people would be given free medical aid. In dispensing medical treatment, the DIA distinguished between deserving and undeserving Aboriginal people. Indian agents were required to swear that a patient was destitute before rendering aid.[65] All the while, DIA employees were repeatedly admonished by the department to reduce medical costs and to refrain from calling doctors to treat "trifling ailments which with medicines and comforts at hand might be treated quite as satisfactorily by an intelligent farming instructor."[66] The drugs purchased by the DIA were the same as those given to the poorest class of white people, and doctors were cautioned to exercise the greatest discretion when sending patients to off-reserve hospitals for treatment.[67] Even those Indian agents who complied with the department's restrictions encountered criticism. Agent Samuel Lucas, after receiving a reprimand for excessive spending, replied with exasperation: "I do not know of any way that I can reduce the cost of medicine or medical attendance. I do not send for the doctor unless he is urgently needed, not on a specified day each month, as was the case before I took charge of the agency."[68]

The federal government did not believe that Treaty 7 had assigned it an obligation to provide medical care. When the DIA was established in 1880, the government made no formal provisions for health care and did not hire medical officers. Indian agents and farm instructors, who had no real medical training or knowledge, were expected to diagnose patients and offer treatment from a medicine chest supplied by the department. A clause in Treaty 6 had referred to a medicine chest and guaranteed aid from the federal government during periods of disease or famine. The federal authorities interpreted this clause narrowly to mean only the provision of supplies.[69] Doctors were employed on a per-call basis and only at the behest of an Indian agent.[70] At treaty payment time, a doctor was present to vaccinate Aboriginal people. Much of this early medical work was designed to prevent the spread of diseases to white communities. Those Aboriginal people who survived the "process of civilization" would be integrated into Euro-Canadian society – a state of affairs that the state thought would be achieved quickly.

Meanwhile, Aboriginal people on their own sought treatment and resources from the state's most visible institution in the West – the NWMP. A NWMP surgeon, Richard Nevitt, was stationed at Fort Macleod when it was built in 1874, and local Aboriginal groups often made use of his medical services. In a letter to his fiancée written on March 8, 1874, Nevitt states: "I am becoming a successful practitioner amongst the simple savages and I think too they all like me, for I am gentle and thoughtful of their feelings just as tho' they were white civilized people. And they, I think, appreciate kindness as much as anyone. When I go to their lodges they give me a smoke always and talk and laugh away in the happiest manner. And any little thing they want done they come to me to get it done for them."[71]

The medical work of the NWMP among Aboriginal peoples was formalized after the signing of Treaty 7. The first medical officer retained on salary by the DIA was the surgeon for the NWMP's Fort Macleod Detachment. His job was to vaccinate Aboriginal people at treaty payment time and to make his services available for all on-call emergencies.[72] In return, the surgeon received six hundred dollars a year. This arrangement came to an end early in 1883, when the NWMP medical officer was relocated to Calgary and his services became too difficult to obtain.[73]

In May 1883 the DIA hired its first full-time physician in the North-West Territories. Historian Maureen Lux found that the DIA took this action not out of concern for the well-being of Aboriginal people but rather in response to petitions from settlers in the region. For instance, in 1882 settlers from Prince Albert, Saskatchewan, wrote that Aboriginal people were "visited with smallpox, scurvy, syphilis, fever, and other loathsome diseases owing to their domestic habits and manner of living."[74] The settlers called on Sir John A. Macdonald, the prime minister of Canada and the superintendent of Indian affairs, to hire a medical superintendent. That person would supervise matters of sanitation on reserves to halt the spread of diseases among Aboriginal peoples, monitor the cross-border movements of Aboriginal peoples, and – most important – prevent the spread of contagious diseases to adjacent white settlements.[75] In response to pressure from settlers and the termination of the DIA's arrangement with the NWMP, Macdonald instructed the Indian commissioner, Edgar Dewdney, to appoint a full-time medical officer. Dr. Francis Xavier Girard was hired at a salary of $1,200 a year.

Originally from Quebec, Girard was living at Fort Macleod when he received his appointment. At first, he was responsible for all of the tribes in southern Alberta, but after several years his responsibilities were reduced.[76] He was placed in charge of only two reserves, the Blood and the Peigan, at a decreased salary of a thousand dollars per year.[77] In her survey of medical officers employed by the DIA in western Canada, Lux presents Girard's career as illustrative of the problems encountered by Aboriginal peoples in their relations with DIA medical officers over the next sixty years.[78] Girard was a patronage appointment, and he used his post with the DIA to support himself while he established a private practice in Fort Macleod. During his visits to a reserve, he was known to visit the Indian agent's house and the Catholic mission. He would then return to Fort Macleod without ever having visited any of the camps.[79] Girard did not possess the confidence of his patients because he did not speak their language, visit the camps regularly, listen to their problems, or visit their homes. Even after it became quite clear that he was not performing his duties adequately, he continued to work for the DIA for almost twenty years.[80]

For the three tribes not supervised by Dr. Girard, the DIA reduced medical costs by hiring doctors on a fee-for-service basis. Doctors received ten dollars for a home visit, one dollar per patient for office visits and prescriptions, and fifty cents a mile for travelling expenses.[81] The practice of hiring medical officers on a part-time basis reflected constant negotiations among federal government officials about appropriate or necessary medical attention for Aboriginal people. This system was invariably determined by two competing concerns: cost and the government's efforts to assimilate Aboriginal peoples. Cost was the most important factor in determining the shape and nature of the health care services provided by the department. Hayter Reed regularly admonished Indian agents to keep medical costs to a minimum. He believed that calling a doctor to attend "sick Indians" was becoming an unnecessary and expensive habit.[82] Officials in the DIA wanted to free land for white settlement and were not interested in aiding what they regarded as a dependent population in need of transformation. DIA administrators believed that if Aboriginal people died in the meantime, it was merely part of the process of going from savagery to civilization.[83]

Hayter Reed believed that Aboriginal people were indolent and lazy, and he instituted policies designed to rid Aboriginal people of these habits. In his view the DIA's task was to make Aboriginal people as much like Euro-Canadians as possible.[84] Duncan Campbell Scott, the deputy superintendent general of Indian affairs from 1913 to 1932, continued Reed's legacy. Scott joined the DIA in 1880, and in 1891 he was placed in charge of the Accountant's Branch, a division of the department that was becoming increasingly important.[85] These two men set the tone within the DIA, which had a mandate to promote self-reliance and individualism among Aboriginal people. Attending physicians were told to directly bill those patients believed to be able to pay, and Aboriginal people were often held responsible for any bills accrued from off-reserve medical facilities.[86] Even during times of recognized medical emergency that affected both white and Aboriginal communities, Indian agents were quick to assure the department that they were not making any undue purchases of medicine or rations.[87] Cost-cutting measures extended to the hiring of physicians, whom the department paid so poorly that it was almost impossible to engage and retain doctors who could provide consistent and regular attendance. The missionary and government systems (if we can call them systems, for the word *system* implies coherence and planning) merged in the 1890s, forming a patchwork of institutions designed to transform Aboriginal people through exposure to Western medicine and Euro-Canadian culture.

Conclusion

The informal healing work that female missionaries performed in mission houses was, to some degree, part of the same network of therapeutic knowledge and caregiving that Aboriginal women made available to their Euro-Canadian counterparts. We can be sure, though, that Euro-Canadian and Aboriginal women viewed their health work very differently. Aboriginal women may very well have helped white women for spiritual reasons, but they did not use their healing work as an opportunity for evangelism. In turn, Euro-Canadian women characterized the healing and caring work they made available to Aboriginal people as emblematic of self-sacrifice, as an outward display of their faith and as part of their service to God and nation. When Euro-Canadian women drew on the curative and caregiving expertise of Aboriginal women, they framed their acceptance as a matter of necessity in the supposedly Wild Canadian West. The only set of therapeutic skills that would not become part of the services that female missionaries offered Aboriginal women was midwifery (for more on this, see Chapter 6). Shared knowledge, healing, and nursing care offer a window on how midwifery and health care produced what Ann Laura Stoler refers to as the intimate frontier. In mission schools the encounters produced by shared domestic space were far more restricted.

The work of missionaries' wives, single female missionaries, the farm women employed by the DIA, and the field matrons appointed by mission societies laid the foundations for many of the public health programs, such as baby shows, that followed in the twentieth century. The evangelical work of missionaries mirrored later efforts by public health and travelling nurses to instruct Aboriginal women in the religion and rules of sanitation and scientific motherhood.[88] Although missionary organizations and white women continued to provide health care on reserves, this work increasingly took place in an institutional environment. The growing involvement of the DIA meant that treatment and nursing care took place in a hospital or school infirmary by Euro-Canadian women with formal nursing training or by female health workers who possessed a great deal of informal experience and knowledge. After 1915, at reserves where cottage hospitals did not exist, the DIA made efforts to hire graduate nurses who could perform both medical and educational roles. The twentieth century witnessed the growing medicalization of reserve space. Most Aboriginal people who had prolonged encounters with biomedicine during this period continued to experience a very feminine version of Western health care.

5
Laying the Foundation

The Work of Nurses, Nursing Sisters, and Female Attendants on Reserves, 1890-1915

During the 1870s and 1880s, the wives of missionaries and female missionaries often provided healing and caregiving in their own homes for local Aboriginal people. The 1890s saw the beginning of a shift in the missions' health work; by 1915, the Anglican, Methodist, and Catholic churches had established hospitals and school infirmaries on reserves. These facilities were staffed by female attendants, including nuns, missionary wives, and formally trained graduate nurses. Euro-Canadian women were instrumental in establishing and maintaining the Western health care system that developed on Treaty 7 reserves. Over time the churches and their mission organizations drew the Department of Indian Affairs (DIA) into funding hospitals and school infirmaries as well as their staff. The medical facilities and health programs launched by the churches during these decades laid the foundation for Indian Health Services (IHS) in the 1920s and 1930s.

The Western therapeutic systems developed by the churches in southern Alberta during the 1890s lacked coherence and varied dramatically between reserves. The colonial health care regime evolved as a patchwork of medical facilities pieced together by individual missionaries and their funding agencies. Some missionaries raised enough money to build cottage hospitals staffed by highly experienced health care workers. Other missionaries made do with whatever funding and staff they could scrape together. One factor remained consistent through the Treaty 7 region – the system relied on the cheap and available labour of female health workers.

As they operated medical facilities and provided ongoing care, Euro-Canadian women were subjected to multiple levels of authority. They were under the supervision of doctors, DIA medical officers, Indian agents, and the church hierarchy. Euro-Canadian women constantly negotiated their duties, levels of patient care, and – more generally – their space in schools, infirmaries, and patients' homes. The physical distance of reserves from urban centres and the infrequent visits of medical officers mitigated some of this control exercised by male supervisors. Even so, whatever freedom these workers enjoyed came at a cost. Euro-Canadian women worked under harsh conditions and were often called on to provide medical treatment that exceeded their training and experience.

The therapeutic labour that Euro-Canadian women performed shaped their relationships with Aboriginal people. In many ways their healing work was similar to the curative and nursing care performed by Aboriginal women. Indeed, the skills of nurses and female medical missionaries were more recognizable to Aboriginal people than those practised by male medical doctors. This meant that Aboriginal people evaluated the healing and nursing work of Euro-Canadian women by the same standards they applied to their own healers. Qualities such as character and dedication figured greatly in their evaluations.[1] The intimate quality of women's nursing and caregiving on reserves allowed some women an opportunity to develop positive cultural understandings. At the same time, however, Euro-Canadian women's interactions with Aboriginal people allowed them to be more effective as agents of the state.

The Growth of Church-Run Health Care Institutions

Church officials in Aboriginal communities quickly noted the ill health that had result from poor economic and social conditions, and they just as quickly came to view the founding of health care facilities as necessary. Reverend Gibbon Stocken, the Anglican missionary among the Tsuu T'ina, was so desperate for a hospital at the reserve that he turned the mission house into a makeshift hospital in the winter of 1892.[2] In a letter to the Church Missionary Society (CMS) in 1893, he describes how much good a hospital and trained staff could do: "Such an institution would provide invaluable aid to the mission because no branch of mission work was so fruitful for good as nursing the sick."[3] At the Peigan Reserve, W.R. Haynes, the resident Anglican missionary, and Miss Garlick, the Anglican missionary at the Victoria Jubilee Home, expressed similar opinions regarding the need for a trained nurse and a hospital. Haynes wrote: "If only we had a hospital and a nurse, or even just a nurse, it would be a great boon, and save many valuable lives. It is very hard on us to have to do our daily work and attend to the sick. We have six other cases of scrofula which have to be carefully attended to and dressed every morning."[4]

In her letter, Miss Garlick describes how happy the Piikani were to receive the meagre medical aid the mission had been able to supply. She calls for a trained nurse and a proper room for the sick because the "greatest needs of these poor people are places for their sick ones."[5] The missionaries' new emphasis on health care was the result of two factors: the ill health they had witnessed during a decade of poverty and starvation and a rising trend in mission work to emphasize good works and welfare services offered by women in the hope of making converts. The Anglican and Catholic churches could not afford to found health care institutions on their own; thus, each mission sought federal government support to establish medical facilities on reserves. Some missionary groups succeeded better than others.

In the 1890s the DIA provided only the most basic medical services to Aboriginal people. By then churches and missionary organizations had been providing Aboriginal people with informal medical aid and nursing care since the late 1870s. Concerned about deteriorating health and the rising costs of health care, missionaries approached the federal government for funding on a mission-by-mission basis. Federal financial support enabled churches and their missions to build small cottage hospitals and school infirmaries. It also allowed them to hire field matrons, graduate nurses, and female nursing attendants. Federal funding created a tight relationship between missionary institutions and the state, thus laying the foundations for what would become IHS.

Some missions were far more effective at acquiring federal patronage than others. It is not known precisely why the government extended them preferential treatment. Perhaps it was the cheap and dedicated labour of the nursing sisters. In the early 1890s, for example, Father Albert Lacombe approached the DIA for money to build a hospital at the Blood Reserve and promised that sisters would run the facility. The DIA supplied the land for the hospital, donated money for its construction, contributed annual maintenance grants, supplied rations for hospital employees, and paid the sisters a modest allowance.[6] Four Sisters of Charity arrived on July 10, 1893, and the hospital was opened in 1894. During the first year, the hospital was run by five sisters: two nursing sisters, one matron, a housekeeper, and a cook.[7] The sisters ran the hospital until September 6, 1954.[8]

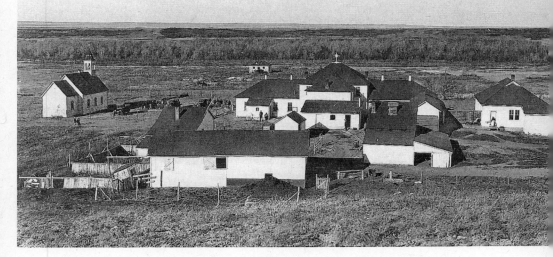

Blood Hospital and pavilions at Standoff, Alberta, n.d. | Courtesy Grey Nuns Archives, Montreal

This Catholic institution encountered fewer difficulties employing and paying staff than many Protestant organizations: most of the sisters who worked at the hospital remained for several decades.

The second hospital to be built in a southern Alberta Aboriginal community received only partial funding from the federal government. Like Father Albert Lacombe, Rev. J.W. Tims approached the DIA in the early 1890s for funding for a medical facility. The Anglican mission started construction of the Blackfoot Hospital in 1894 with funding from a variety of sources: the federal government, the Anglican Church of Canada, and the Toronto Women's Auxiliary. The federal money was insufficient, and although the hospital was built in 1894, it was not completed, furnished, or even occupied until 1897.[9] The building had two wards – one for women and children, the other for men – with eight beds in each, as well as a bathroom, a dispensary, a kitchen, a hall, a pantry, and staff quarters for seven.[10]

Stable financial support from the Toronto Women's Auxiliary was crucial to the success of the Blackfoot Hospital. It would not have been finished without its support, for it was the auxiliary that supplied the

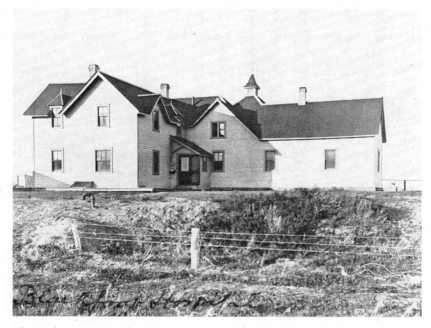

The Anglican-run Blackfoot Hospital, late 1890s. | Courtesy Glenbow Archives NA-1773-17

linens and furnishings for the nurses' quarters, paid the salaries of three nurses or nursing assistants, and provided an annual maintenance grant.[11] This organization would continue to support the Blackfoot Hospital, even forming a Blackfoot Hospital Committee, which met annually until 1923, when the federal government used band funds to erect a new thirty-five-bed hospital.[12] Without the financial and moral support of women's auxiliaries, few missions in the Treaty 7 region would have had the medical facilities they did, however inadequate they were.

    The Blood and Blackfoot hospitals were the only facilities in the Treaty 7 area during this period to receive this degree of largesse from the DIA. Other missions made do with sporadic funding from Ottawa on a situation-by-situation basis. This money was earmarked for equipment, minor maintenance, and nurses' salaries. None of this funding was long-term, and missions at the Peigan, Sarcee, and Stoney reserves were compelled to scramble for money from the churches, women's auxiliaries, and the Women's Missionary Society (WMS) of the Methodist Church of Canada. Anglican women's auxiliaries and the WMS raised money to pay for nurses, equipment, medical supplies, and furniture. They also donated clothing, toys, games, and treats for the children. Most often it was women's missionary organizations that paid the salaries of female health workers.

The Anglican missions provide a perfect example of the complicated and precarious financial circumstances faced by most church-run health care institutions in the Treaty 7 area in the late nineteenth and early twentieth centuries. The Anglican missionary at the Peigan Reserve succeeded in cobbling together enough money from the Anglican Church and various women's auxiliaries to build a small cottage hospital, the Victoria Home Hospital, near the Anglican residential school. This facility suffered from unstable funding and was often without a nurse. An example of the piecemeal funding available from the DIA was the twenty-five-dollars-a-month nursing assistant's salary it agreed to pay in 1915. Shortly after the nursing assistant was hired, however, the DIA stopped paying for her salary.[13] The Victoria Home Hospital served mainly as a school infirmary that permitted caregivers to keep sick children separate from their families.[14] Reports from the Victoria Home Hospital reveal that most students sent there were treated for tuberculosis. Once the students improved, they were returned to the school.[15] This hospital closed in February 1919 because of inadequate funding.[16]

The Anglican mission at the Blood Reserve faced a similar state of affairs. The Anglican missionary at the reserve was especially keen to build a hospital that could compete with the Catholic one. Indeed, the Anglicans were fiercely jealous of the Catholic hospital and the funding the federal government bestowed on it. The Anglican missionary for the Kainai succeeded in raising money for a building from the Anglican Church, the Society for the Promotion of Christian Knowledge, and various women's auxiliaries. Built in 1896, this short-lived institution did not have a nurse until May 1900, when a small grant from the Huron Women's Auxiliary paid for the nurse's salary and the final furnishings for the building.[17] Even after the auxiliary donated money, however, the facility remained open only part of the year because the Anglicans could not secure a nurse who was willing to work so hard and remain at such an isolated post.[18]

The Anglican mission among the Tsuu T'ina was underfunded even more severely than the missions at the Peigan and Blood reserves. Despite repeated attempts, the missionary was unable to raise enough money to build a hospital. The Sarcee Residential School was instead served by a small school infirmary.[19] The reserve's proximity to Calgary made it unlikely that a hospital would ever be built. The Anglican mission at the Sarcee Reserve periodically obtained the services of a graduate nurse, who served as both nurse and residential school matron.[20] Her salary was paid by one of the women's auxiliaries. Not until 1915 did the DIA provide funding for a full-time trained nurse, and only after an inspector's report revealed gravely high rates of tubercular infection.

The Methodists were the last mission organization to establish a hospital in southern Alberta, this one among the Nakoda. It received very little funding from the federal government. The life of this small cottage hospital was tightly linked to McDougall Residential School, which it served, and to WMS funding. It was erected in 1906. Throughout its existence, the hospital had only one staff member, a female missionary with nursing training, whose salary and board were paid by the WMS.[21] Sometimes the nurse was helped by a field matron, who was also employed by the WMS. The hospital accommodated eight patients. In 1908, tents were erected to house twenty-eight beds that would serve as an isolation ward for TB patients.[22] Students from the school were the institution's main patrons. This facility closed along with the school in 1910.[23]

Between 1890 and 1915, the location of medical care at the Blood and Blackfoot reserves gradually shifted from domestic settings to more clinical surroundings. In part this was the result of DIA doctors' increasing reluctance to provide care in Aboriginal people's own homes. Doctors insisted that reserve residents come to the hospital to be cared for properly.[24] This approach was strongly supported by DIA officials, who agreed with DIA physicians that Aboriginal people did not follow medical instructions, lived in unsanitary conditions, and allowed medicine men to interfere in recovery.[25] At the Sarcee, Peigan, and Stoney reserves, the school infirmaries established by the missions did not alter the location of Western medical treatment. The infirmaries remained places in which students were kept until they could be returned to the boarding school (i.e., instead of being sent home). During their monthly visits, the DIA doctors continued to treat residents either at dispensaries located near the Indian agent's office or, in the case of an extreme emergency, in the homes of Aboriginal people. The DIA did not recognize any formal responsibility for providing Western health care for Aboriginal people. In addition, department officials believed that the department was already giving the churches and their missionary organizations more than enough money to provide these services in its place. Unfortunately, ill health and poverty continued to be problems on reserves in southern Alberta.

The bureaucracy of the DIA's Medical Branch was slow to evolve. One of the first steps in its development was the appointment of Dr. Peter H. Bryce in 1904 as the first general medical superintendent responsible for

Indian health. Bryce had come to the attention of the DIA when he served as secretary of Ontario's Provincial Board of Health. As secretary, he had repeatedly and publicly expressed his concern about the DIA's failure to deal appropriately with outbreaks of contagious diseases on reserves.[26] In a politically astute move, Clifford Sifton, minister of the interior, appointed Bryce as chief medical officer for the Departments of the Interior and Indian Affairs. In other words, he would be responsible for health inspections, quarantines, and the promotion of proper sanitation and hygiene among both immigrants and Aboriginal people.[27] Bryce's appointment propelled minor changes on reserves, for he believed strongly that the DIA needed to reorganize and directly manage medical services to control and suppress contagious diseases. Under Bryce the DIA's health efforts focused on public health, communicable diseases, and recording birth and death rates. Bryce was fired, however, by Duncan Campbell Scott in 1913.

Bryce thought that the state should play a direct role in social reform and take steps to improve Aboriginal health and welfare. In 1907 he submitted a report about conditions in western Canada's residential schools.[28] This report did not provoke immediate change; indeed, not until 1909, when Duncan Campbell Scott was appointed the first superintendent of education, would standards be imposed relating to the construction and maintenance of residential schools.[29] Some of Bryce's proposed reforms were instituted – for example, tents were raised for the treatment of tubercular patients, and health circulars were instituted. However, two of the great hallmarks of Indian administration – efficiency and economy – continued: "Scott would remain the greatest champion of both throughout his tenure with the DIA."[30]

Under Scott the DIA began wresting control of Aboriginal health care from the churches. There were two main reasons for this development. First, Scott was concerned about alarming reports of ill health in residential schools. Historian Maureen Lux notes that the DIA was committed to protecting the "department's pre-eminent institutions for social and cultural change," and disease drastically reduced the effectiveness of the schools' civilizing program.[31] Bryce revealed in a report to the Canadian Tuberculosis Association in 1906 that the government's annual expenditure of $2 million on education was largely being wasted, given that 75 percent of residential-school graduates died before they turned eighteen.[32] Second, the churches, according to the DIA, seemed unable to manage the schools and hospitals properly. Instead of viewing the grants that the DIA had given to the churches as inadequate, department officials contended that the problem lay with the churches' shoddy management practices. Bryce believed that these concerns needed to be addressed by introducing regular health inspections, publishing hygiene manuals for staff and students, employing properly trained medical workers at residential schools, and (as noted earlier) erecting small tent hospitals adjacent to boarding schools for TB patients.[33] Concerns about the poor health of residential-school students and the supposedly incompetent administration of missionary organizations sparked an expansion of state-run health services after 1915.

Training Female Attendants

Not all of the Euro-Canadian women who provided curative services on reserves in southern Alberta possessed formal nursing training. Especially before 1900, only some of the women working for the Anglican Church were nurses who had graduated with two or three years' training in teaching hospitals. Often those women who did possess formal training came from outside Canada.[34] This was not unusual, considering that the first training hospital in Canada, the General and Marine Hospital in St. Catharines, Ontario, was not opened until 1874.[35] In Alberta the first nurse training program was offered at Medicine Hat General in August 1894. Only two women entered the program in the first year. That same year Calgary General opened its training program with only one student.[36] Misericordia Hospital and Edmonton General opened their nursing programs in 1907 and 1908, respectively.[37] It is unlikely that any of these women ever worked on reserves in southern Alberta, given the demand for trained nurses in the region. Few of the trained medical missionary women during this period were local: most came from eastern Canada or Britain. This was especially true of the Grey Nuns at the Blood Hospital, who blended their nursing care with the Catholic faith and were reluctant to allow Protestant or even Roman Catholic lay women to intrude on their religious community.

Those women who did not possess formal nursing credentials acquired their nursing skills informally, that is, through experience and practice. Euro-Canadian women's unofficial training often translated into considerable expertise in terms of both care and the medical assistance they could provide Aboriginal people.[38] Although Protestant female missionaries and the wives of missionaries who offered medical services at the mission houses did not have nursing training, they were able to provide bedside care, administer first aid, and oversee basic social services. The Grey Nuns likewise lacked formal nursing credentials, but they had a long history of running Catholic hospitals and providing nursing assistance to the poor and the sick.[39] The Hôpital Notre-Dame in Montreal, run by the Grey Nuns, was the first hospital in Canada to offer instruction in French, beginning in 1898.[40]

The Anglicans found it difficult to recruit and retain qualified nursing personnel for their institutions. Unlike their Roman Catholic counterparts, Anglican missionary societies did not have a pool of experienced and dedicated nursing sisters to draw from. The staff at an Anglican hospital often consisted of a single trained nurse. There were times when the Women's Auxiliary of the Anglican Church had no choice but to hire women who lacked nursing certification. One example is Jane Megarry, the matron at the Blackfoot Hospital, who during the First World War had been enrolled in the nursing program at the Royal Jubilee Hospital in Victoria, BC, but who left before her training was completed. The Anglican hospitals at the Peigan and Blood reserves often had to shut their doors because of staff shortages. Even the Blackfoot Hospital, the longest-lasting and best-funded Anglican hospital in the Treaty 7 area, often had only one graduate nurse on staff. That hospital was completed in 1894, but suitable personnel were unavailable until Isabel Turner – a graduate nurse who had been in charge of the dispensary at a hospital in Erie, Pennsylvania – and her sister Alice applied for positions. Alice Turner possessed no professional nursing training but did have a great deal of personal experience as housekeeper, cook, and night nurse.[41] The Turner sisters worked in southern Alberta for less than two years.

The inability of Protestant organizations to retain staff was reflected in the erratic management and record keeping of individual Anglican institutions. At the Blackfoot Hospital, for example, Dr. Rose's wife served as administrator from 1901 to 1904, when she left her post because of overwork and exhaustion. Before and after her tenure, the names of administrative personnel are not specified in DIA records. Female nursing attendants performed most patient care and treatment and generally maintained the institution, but it is unclear who requested supplies and submitted monthly reports to the DIA. Limited evidence suggests that female Protestant missionaries reported to the person in charge of that particular mission, who in turn submitted medical reports to the DIA. The Blackfoot Hospital did not keep consistent medical records and reports. In 1913, J.H. Gooderham, the Indian agent at the Blood Reserve, reprimanded Reverend Stocken for failing to submit the proper paperwork to his office.[42] Frequent staff changes made it impossible for the Anglicans to keep accurate and detailed records of who had attended the hospital and who had used the dispensary and for what reasons.

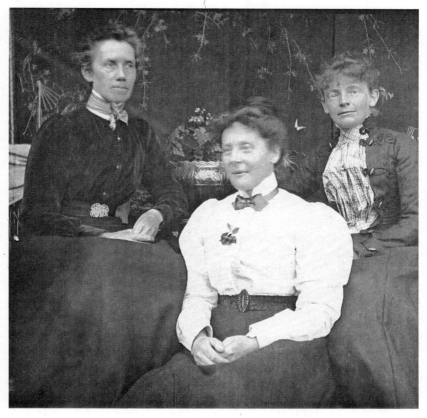

The nursing staff at the Blackfoot Hospital, late 1890s. *L-R:* Miss Easom, Miss Isabel Turner, and Miss Alice Turner. | Courtesy Glenbow Archives NA-4928-23

At the Catholic Blood Hospital, the situation was entirely different. The position of sister superior was rotated every three years, and the sister chosen for the job was always picked from among staff with experience working at Aboriginal missions. Because women who had worked at the institution for many years were usually chosen, the Catholic missions provided a continuity in service that Protestant missions could not match. The sister superior was responsible for the day-to-day operations of the hospital: ordering supplies, ensuring that repairs and maintenance were carried out, dealing with the Indian agent, and supervising the staff of the nursing sisters and the handyman, who was usually an Aboriginal man from the reserve. Monthly records of who used the hospital and why are available, but they only tell us each patient's name, illness, and number of days spent in the hospital, along with whether she or he was cured. Catholic-run institutions, while they kept relatively thorough records, were as silent as the Anglican ones regarding the day-to-day work that nurses performed. To investigate the healing work that women performed, a careful reading of the sources is required.

Nursing Work in Hospitals and Dispensaries

Those historians who have looked at the medical work of Euro-Canadian missionary women among Aboriginal peoples have largely ignored the curative labours of the women hired by the DIA.[43] The informal medical aid and bedside care provided by missionary women during the late nineteenth and early twentieth centuries was comparable to many of the tasks later performed by trained nurses engaged by the DIA to work in reserve hospitals, dispensaries, temporary facilities, and people's homes. Most significantly, these Euro-Canadian women performed analogous educational or public health roles. The religious evangelism of female missionaries was slowly supplanted by the doctrine of public health propounded by graduate and travelling nurses – so slowly, indeed, that the shift is difficult to trace today. Lay female health workers did not outnumber medical missionaries on Treaty 7 reserves until the mid-1920s, and in some institutions – such as the Blood Hospital – women with strong religious affiliations continued to blend religion with Western biomedicine until well into the 1950s.

Scholars who have investigated the impact of Western medicine on Aboriginal peoples in Canada tend to view the Euro-Canadians who provided medical services as indistinguishable. That is, historians often assume that the care offered by women was exactly the same as that offered by men. For instance, James Waldram, D. Ann Herring, and T. Kue Young's book – probably the most extensive examination of medicine and Aboriginal peoples in Canada from pre-contact to the present – does not take account of the nursing and caregiving work of Euro-Canadian women.[44] According to the authors, medical services on reserves were provided by male medical professionals. This oversight is in part a result of the weight assigned to men and doctors in the primary sources, but it is also a result of failing to include gender as a category of analysis when looking at the colonizers.

Canadian scholars of nursing history have begun to redress this gap in the literature. Two noteworthy articles investigate the role that public health nurses played on reserves in western Canada. One is by Laurie

Meijer Drees and Lesley McBain, the other is by Kathryn McPherson.[45] Both articles deal only with the post-1930 period and do not discuss the genesis of health care in western Canada. Even so, they offer a framework for analyzing the place of Euro-Canadian women on reserves. All three authors found that as Euro-Canadian women attempted to address health concerns in Aboriginal communities and attend to local needs, their identities as nurses, as women, and as employees of the state came into conflict. In their efforts to make a strange and chronically underfunded system effective, they were forced to re-evaluate their position and place.[46]

Historians have done a much more thorough job when it comes to examining the roles of female missionaries in Canada. They agree that the work of Euro-Canadian women was central to the churches' Christianizing and civilizing efforts. The popular literature of the late nineteenth and early twentieth centuries depicted mission work as a masculine endeavour.[47] Yet recent studies have found that the labour of Euro-Canadian women was central to supporting and maintaining mission work. In the beginning, women volunteered their time and raised money for mission societies at home. They later provided a steady supply of cheap labour for increasingly important social welfare, teaching, and health care tasks.[48] Although missionary work was viewed as a socially acceptable alternative to marriage, women's missionary work was constrained by perceptions regarding appropriate work for women.[49] In the field they served in ways considered suitable for women – as nurses, teachers, field matrons, caregivers, housekeepers, and so on.[50] Women's work in these areas was one of the few means available for Euro-Canadians to reach Aboriginal communities that showed little interest in converting to Christianity.

The Euro-Canadian women who worked at Treaty 7 reserves performed a wide range of therapeutic, social service, and educational functions. At the hospitals and schools, medical missionaries cared for patients, oversaw treatments, ran the dispensary, and prepared meals for outpatients. Those women who worked beyond institutional boundaries, providing care in Aboriginal people's homes, had to offer a broader range of medical services. Besides carrying out their medical responsibilities, they were expected to provide domestic and religious instruction. Many of the women who worked at reserves were unprepared for the working conditions and cultural differences. Still, some of them found the work rewarding and forged long-lasting friendships with Aboriginal women.

In most cases, however, white women saw the provision of Western medicine as an opportunity to educate Aboriginal women about Euro-Canadian culture and values. For example, it was extremely important to provide aseptic conditions in reserve hospitals, and female health care workers saw this as an opportunity to teach Aboriginal women that "cleanliness was next to godliness."[51] During the late nineteenth and early twentieth centuries, Western medicine served as the "go-between that linked the two poles [of social and moral] reform both symbolically and practically."[52] Thus, as historian Myra Ruthedale persuasively argues, "cleanliness was next to godliness because cleanliness was visible and belief in Christianity was certainly much less tangible."[53] For Euro-Canadian female missionaries, observable bodily and domestic transformations were closely linked to the spiritual development of Aboriginal women and served as concrete measures of their progress.

The rudimentary conditions that prevailed in reserve hospitals often interfered with the ability of female health care workers to promote cleanliness. In a letter to Mrs. Cummings, the head of the Toronto Women's Auxiliary, Isabel Turner, a health worker at the Blackfoot Hospital, complained bitterly about the lack of a proper room to bath patients.[54] She was forced to use the dispensary for this task, which interfered with the staff's ability to treat outpatients. The poor water supply exacerbated the situation and created considerable difficulties for hospital personnel. Isabel and Alice Turner found it hard to keep the facility clean, and their housekeeping duties were so heavy that they hired outside help, which they paid for out of their own pockets. In contrast, the sisters at the Catholic Blood Hospital rotated housekeeping chores.

Another significant obstacle to patient care was that reserve hospitals were poorly constructed and poorly planned. A report from a contractor who inspected the Catholic Blood Hospital in 1924 provides gruesome detail about the building's plumbing. Waste of all sorts was emptied into a cesspit behind the hospital, and the interior plumbing was so poor that the bathtubs either did not empty or filled up with a foul-smelling effluent.[55] The hospital's small water tank did not supply enough water for four departments; as a result, most of the water for the hospital had to be hauled from the river in barrels.[56] These conditions made the sisters' work so arduous that when the hospital was renovated in 1928, the reverend general commented specifically on how much the sisters' work would be reduced by improved conditions.[57]

On top of their housekeeping duties, female health workers made meals available – not only to the hospital's inpatients but also to outpatients, patients' family members, and dispensary cases, as well as to certain special cases. In fact, it seems that one of the main functions of the hospital (and of some schools) was to provide meals to so-called deserving reserve

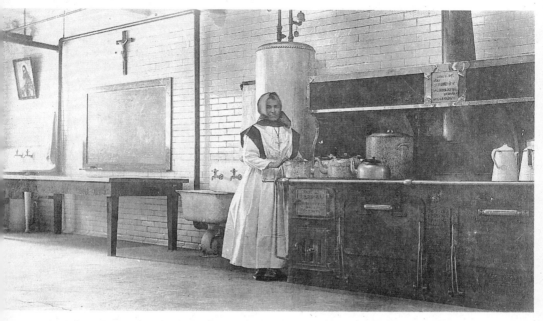

Grey Nun working in the kitchen at the Blood Hospital, n.d. | Courtesy Grey Nuns Archives, Montreal

residents. At one point, W. J. Dilworth, the Indian agent at the Blood Reserve, suggested closing down the Blood Hospital, for it seemed to him that its main purpose was to serve as a soup kitchen rather than a medical facility.[58] For female mission staff, a soup kitchen was desirable because it reflected a shared and gendered perception among hospital workers and reserve residents that good, healthy food was necessary and that the provision of it was something – in keeping with the dominant discourse of the day – that women were well placed to give.

At the Blood Hospital, two or three outpatients came in for several meals a day. One was Mrs. Calf Child, who came to the hospital every chance she had and told the nurses she had "a little bird inside of her that made her hungry and must be fed."[59] The Blackfoot Hospital hired extra staff to help with all the cooking and baking that needed to be done.[60] In 1914 Jane Megarry described the meals they fed visitors at the hospital: "We gave them a warm meal when they arrived, a bowl of beef stew with plenty of vegetables in it. Homemade bread and a cup of tea."[61] The hospitals also sent food to sick people who lived at home. In 1911 Miss Murray, the matron at the Blackfoot Hospital, indicated that most of her time was spent treating outpatients and that as a result the hospital was kept very busy sending meals to the camp two or three times a day.[62] To keep up with the demand for fresh food, the Blood and Blackfoot hospitals kept gardens and cows.[63] Reserve residents were clearly using the hospitals as a lifeline at a time of dwindling local resources, insufficient rations, ill health, and starvation.

The hospitals provided short-term care for residential schoolchildren and were extremely important in this capacity. Reserve doctors used the hospitals as a means to temporarily provide sick and malnourished students with better food. The treatments doctors prescribed were often directly related to the inadequate nutritional regime provided in residential schools. Female health care workers at the hospital were instructed to feed schoolchildren eggnog, fresh milk, and eggs to "improve their constitutions."[64] When students gained weight and seemed to be recovering, they were returned to the school. But reserve hospitals and school infirmaries were a temporary solution and did not prevent the spread of infectious diseases. Indeed, John Milloy's study of residential schools shows that the poorly constructed buildings, crowded living conditions, insufficient food, and poor clothing made them breeding grounds for contagious diseases.[65] Conditions at some church-run schools were so poor that even missionaries cautioned parents against sending their children to them. Marchmont Ing, the Methodist missionary in charge of the Stoney Reserve in the 1890s and early 1900s, warned Nakoda parents about the danger the McDougall Residential School posed to the health of their children. Shortly afterwards, the school's principal complained about Ing, who was forthwith removed from his post and stationed among a white congregation in Calgary, where he would be less disruptive.[66]

Another important aspect of patient care was keeping patients occupied while they recuperated. Since so many inpatients were children, this task was doubly challenging. Requests from female hospital workers to women's auxiliaries for necessities such as clothing, medicine, and material for making bandages also listed games, toy soldiers, blocks, checkers, picture books, and magazines.[67] Alma Booth recalled that she had kept the patients at the Blackfoot Hospital amused by looking at magazines and scrapbooks, playing games, and reading books. Alice Rumney, a nurse at the Blackfoot Hospital, always sang to her patients and encouraged them to sing hymns with her.[68] Rumney's use of hymns to occupy her patients serves as a reminder that such activities always served a dual purpose – entertainment and proselytization.

Besides caring for patients, the graduate nurses, nursing sisters, nursing assistants, and female missionaries performed educational tasks. Home visits remained an important weapon in the arsenal of female mission workers because they allowed Euro-Canadian women to combine evangelical work with domestic instruction. This blending of religion with lessons on housekeeping and child care was an extension of the healing and nursing work that Euro-Canadian women provided at mission houses and in residential schools.[69] Mission staff also hoped that when Aboriginal people stayed in hospital they would witness first-hand the benefits of domestic hygiene.

Church-run institutions came to represent both progress and Western culture. Female health care workers believed that their work in hospitals, dispensaries, and school infirmaries served as an example to Aboriginal women of the benefits to be gained from European culture. Nurses thought that exposure to the facilities would induce Aboriginal people, especially women, to adopt the same precepts of cleanliness and order as had been established in church-run institutions.[70] For Euro-Canadian women, housework and domestic labour symbolized "social values, segregating dirt from hygiene, order from disorder, meaning from confusion."[71] These values were perceived as being absent from Aboriginal society. It followed that through domestic labour and the transformation of home Aboriginal women would make civilization and order from savagery and disorder.

The DIA's funding for church-run hospitals and dispensaries was often parsimonious; even so, the federal government fully endorsed the ideological agenda of the missionaries' health initiatives. The DIA believed that Aboriginal people who did not make use of Western medical facilities were showing a blatant disregard for the health and well-being of their communities and children. The department's view of proper parenting, especially mothering, reflected the adoption of a broader ideological concept in Canadian society at the turn of the century — scientific motherhood. Historian Cynthia Comacchio, who has studied scientific motherhood in Canada, argues that medical professionals believed that mothers were constrained by their "ignorance [of proper childrearing, which] could be remedied only through expert tutoring and supervision." For Aboriginal women, this need for expert tutelage was seen as doubly necessary.[72]

The DIA did not agree with the approach that Aboriginal people, especially women, took to raising their children. Department officials believed that Aboriginal people were careless parents. In an annual report submitted to the DIA, Agent Samuel Lucas of the Sarcee Reserve writes that Aboriginal women "[did] not exercise the least control over their children, they are allowed to go in or out, sick or well, during the most inclement weather, often insufficiently clad."[73] Because of the flawed connections that child welfare campaigners drew between poverty and poor parenting, Aboriginal women were subjected to harsh criticism by the DIA and health care workers more generally. Aboriginal mothers were blamed for the ill health of their children. The DIA used so-called poor parenting as an opportunity to rationalize its failure to substantively address living conditions on reserves and as a means to legitimize the ever increasing intrusion of the state into the homes of Aboriginal people. This work laid the foundations for the labour of nurses after 1915, when religion was replaced by the gospel of public health. The manner in which public health nurses approached their work with Aboriginal mothers was greatly influenced by the explosion of literature on parenting in the 1920s. Experts published works on childrearing that sought to teach parents to replace "common sense as the final determinant of effective child-rearing strategies with scientific knowledge" to produce better healthier children.[74] Given the ill health in Aboriginal communities, public health nurses saw the implementation of this child care advice as central to the assimilation of Treaty 7 peoples.

But much of the nursing care performed by graduate nurses, nursing sisters, and nursing assistants in reserve hospitals, temporary medical stations, and even the homes of Aboriginal people revolved around caring for patients with chronic illnesses. This work largely involved treating symptoms associated with respiratory illnesses such as TB and eye problems such as trachoma. In 1890 the death rate among the prairie Aboriginal population was 90 per 1,000, and TB and related illnesses accounted for two-thirds of those deaths.[75] Female health workers at hospital dispensaries were kept busy by patients who came to have their tubercular and scrofulous sores cleaned and dressed daily.[76] With the exception of residential school students, this treatment took place mainly on an outpatient basis because few reserve residents consented to remain as hospital inpatients.

The resistance of reserve residents to prolonged hospital stays was the result of several factors. First, Aboriginal people found the hospital to be a sterile and institutional place. They were accustomed to being surrounded by family and friends during times of illness. Second, reserve residents refused to sleep or stay in buildings where people had died. At the Blackfoot Reserve, even after the Anglican-run hospital was opened, a dying woman was kept at the mission house to be looked after by Mrs. Stocken, the missionary's wife, because "hopeless cases [could not] be admitted to the hospital, the Indians being so superstitious."[77] Finally, hospital conditions

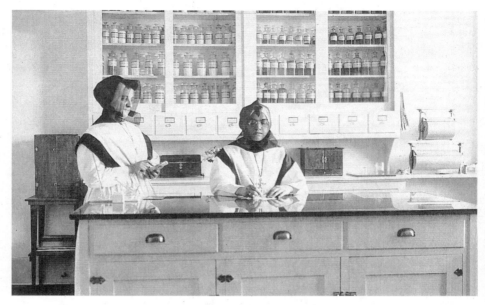

Grey Nuns working in the dispensary at the Blood Hospital, 1930. | Courtesy Grey Nuns Archives, Montreal

rarely met the standards expected by Aboriginal people, who often chose to attend off-reserve facilities, where they received better care and had access to the latest technology and treatments.[78]

Much of the day-to-day healing work performed by Euro-Canadians therefore took place at the hospital dispensary or near the Indian agent's house. There were 6 inpatients but 308 dispensary cases at the Blood Hospital in June 1911; there were 18 inpatients but 327 dispensary cases in November 1912.[79] The Blackfoot Hospital housed 85 inpatients in 1897-98 but handled 2,139 dispensary cases. Hospital staff attended 72 inpatients and 630 dispensary cases in 1905; they dealt with 51 inpatients and 466 dispensary cases in 1911.[80] The decline in the number of dispensary cases at the Blackfoot Hospital after 1898 was related directly to the relocation of the mission and residential school to a new site at the reserve. Most people who attended the Blackfoot Hospital dispensary had been either students of the residential school or were members of their families. Alice Turner described the importance of the hospital dispensary to her community in a letter to the Toronto Women's Auxiliary: "The dispensary is open from early morning till late at night and the Indians very few of whom have clocks, come at all hours for their daily dressings."[81] In her survey of DIA health care institutions in western Canada, historian Maureen Lux found that Aboriginal people eagerly used reserve dispensaries while the hospital beds remained empty.[82]

The labour of Euro-Canadian women encompassed a range of responsibilities. The typical male medical officer worked part-time, and he usually lived not at the reserve but in the town or city. Euro-Canadian women who worked at Treaty 7 reserves were therefore forced to take on responsibilities that did not normally fall within the boundaries of nursing practice. Nurses were expected to make diagnoses and carry out treatments more commonly handled by physicians. Some of the curative duties carried out by nurses required considerable skill and experience. One of the tasks assigned to nurses in residential schools, especially after 1910, was administering tuberculin and saline injections to students suffering from TB. The school nurses recorded detailed observations of students' reactions for the medical officer.[83] Female health workers were sometimes called on to set broken bones and other serious injuries.

Physical isolation and the immediate needs of patients required female attendants to exceed their usual duties. Most of the dispensary work at hospitals was undertaken by graduate nurses or nursing sisters. Reporting symptoms to a doctor and then waiting for him to appear was not a reasonable alternative, especially for reserve residents who required immediate treatment. The attending doctor for the hospital usually lived some distance from the reserve and visited once or twice a week. Dr. Rose, the medical officer hired by the CMS to attend the Blackfoot Hospital twice a week, lived five miles away in Gleichen, where he had a private practice. Besides serving as medical officers, DIA doctors often had private practices in Euro-Canadian communities. Others owned businesses, ran ranches, or held public office.[84]

Nurses often had to provide a wide range of medical services without a physician's immediate supervision. K. Margaret Laing was hired by the Methodist WMS to work at the Morley Hospital. She had received her nursing training at the General Hospital in Guelph, Ontario, before spending a year at the Methodist National Training School in 1900. Her first posting was in Kanazawa, Japan, from 1900 to 1905. She was stationed among the Nakoda from 1906 to 1910. In 1910 she requested reassignment and was sent to the Aboriginal hospital at Port Simpson. She retired from the mission field in 1921.

At the Morley Hospital, Laing examined patients, made diagnoses, and decided on appropriate treatments.[85] During her tenure at the reserve, she treated venereal diseases, set broken arms, and examined all children under five for TB.[86] On one visit to a woman's house, she examined a patient who was in considerable pain. Before she could complete her examination, the family forced her to stop. Before she could proceed with her work, she needed the consent of the patient and her family, which was not forthcoming. Aboriginal people did not blindly submit to the examinations of Western health care workers: white medicine and its practitioners were subjected to the same standards that Aboriginal people applied to their own medicine. If they did not have confidence that a treatment was needed or would succeed, they would not subscribe to it.[87] In this particular case, Laing instead gave the family medicine and directions and left.[88] Although she worked in the small hospital attached to the Morley schools, much of her medical work took place in the homes of Nakoda residents, who were scattered throughout the reserve. Because the help of a doctor would have been difficult to acquire, Laing was compelled to rely on her own knowledge and skills to deal with most medical situations. In a letter to *Missionary Outlook,* she emphasized the importance of her work to her financial backers in eastern Canada and observed that she was the only Western health care worker living at the reserve and that the doctor in charge lived in Calgary.[89]

Religious organizations recognized the therapeutic and economic value of nurses' work. The visits of DIA medical officers were unpredictable, expensive, and sometimes of limited healing effect. Regardless of whether they were formally trained, nurses were a solution to the financial constraints under which church-run institutions operated. For instance, the fathers at St. Joseph's Industrial School (the Dunbow School) east of High River, Alberta, complained that no benefits had come from the formal, hurried, and intermittent physician's visits. As an affordable alternative, the fathers suggested that medical decisions at Dunbow be left in the hands of Sister Kelly, the school's sister superior.[90] Most likely the fathers preferred to keep medical decisions within the community and under their control. Sister Kelly, although not a graduate nurse, knew first aid, was a trained pharmacist, had years of hospital experience, and was skilled in ordinary diagnoses and the treatment of simple illnesses.[91] After lengthy negotiations with the DIA, it was agreed that medical services at Dunbow would be retained on an on-call basis – a decision, moreover, left to Sister Kelly's discretion.[92]

It seems that all Treaty 7 reserves confronted similar health and living conditions throughout the period, regardless of the form Western health care took in their communities. For instance, in 1904 a major smallpox epidemic struck every Aboriginal community in southern Alberta. The Blood and Blackfoot reserves had hospitals, yet both communities suffered significant reductions in their populations. That year, the death rate at the Blackfoot Reserve was 100 per 1,000, while at the Blood Reserve it was 110 per 1,000. Although the statistics available for the Piikani are incomplete, their death rate that year was considerably lower, at 25 per 1,000.[93] The reason for this discrepancy is unknown. Statistics such as these suggest that health in Aboriginal communities was directly linked to material conditions rather than to the reluctance of Aboriginal people to use Western medicine – or at least the Western medicine that was available at their reserves. That ill health persisted despite the presence of Western health facilities suggests that the problem lay elsewhere. Studies by Mary-Ellen Kelm and Maureen Lux have dispelled the myth that Aboriginal bodies were inherently sickly. Instead, Kelm and Lux contend that there is a direct correlation between morbidity and mortality rates and poor rations, insufficient clothing, inadequate housing, diminishing local resources, declining access to hunting and gathering activities, and the federal government's harsh governance.[94]

Negotiating Work, Place, and Patient Care

The autonomy that Euro-Canadian women were extended at reserve health care facilities sometimes led to conflict between DIA medical officers and female nursing attendants. Although the latter might have been in charge in the absence of doctors, female health workers were ultimately expected to acquiesce to male physicians' authority. But given the infrequency of doctor's visits, this adherence to the medical hierarchy was not always strictly followed at reserve hospitals, and this became a source of conflict. On one occasion Isabel Turner, the nurse in charge at the Blackfoot Hospital, refused to help Dr. James Lafferty perform an operation because she disagreed with his assessment of the patient's condition.[95] This disagreement was part of a broader negotiation over the rights of doctors to ultimate control over church-run hospitals and the medical missionaries who worked in them. In 1899 Lafferty protested to the DIA his lack of authority when it came to admitting patients to the Blackfoot Hospital and the infirmary at the Old Sun Residential School.[96] Lafferty also complained bitterly about not being kept apprised of the medical procedures being applied and the decisions being made in his absence. The department ruled that although the hospital had been established by the Anglican Church through private donations, it was now being maintained by government grants. It was, therefore, a state facility under the supervision of DIA officers.

All admissions, treatments, and discharges needed to be approved by the medical officer in charge.[97] This decision was emblematic of the declining autonomy that mission facilities faced in this era.

The situation was more complicated at the Roman Catholic hospital. Besides the constraints they faced as women, the sisters were subject to the church's authority. In January 1913 the bishop of St. Albert reprimanded the sisters at the Blood Hospital for failing to follow the DIA doctor's directions regarding the admission and discharge of patients. The bishop understood that the sisters had in the past possessed more authority in the administration of the hospital. But he also observed that this was no longer the case and that the nuns must conform to how other hospitals operated.[98] The sisters clearly answered to multiple levels of authority. They were subject not only to their superiors at the hospital and within their own order but also to the hierarchy of the Catholic Church.

Nurses, nursing sisters, and female health workers also had to negotiate the terms of patient care with medical officers and department officials. For example, in January 1913 Dr. O.C. Edwards discharged an old woman from the Blood Hospital on the grounds that he could do nothing for her and that the hospital was not intended to house incurables. The sisters disagreed with Edwards' decision and reported it to the Indian agent, who in turn wrote to the DIA requesting permission to readmit the woman. Permission was granted, and the old woman was returned to the hospital, where she died several days later.[99] Female health workers often perceived their role as being at odds with the mandate laid out by the DIA's medical officers.

The nurses at the Blackfoot Hospital and the sisters at the Blood Hospital made it a practice to allow patients' families – especially mothers of young patients – to remain at the hospital with them. Hospital records show mothers being admitted and fed alongside their children, and vice versa. The DIA and its medical officers made repeated attempts to end this practice, but throughout this period female health workers continued to allow family members to remain with loved ones.[100] Indeed, notwithstanding official attempts to disallow this practice, Dr. Stone unofficially authorized it in 1931 in a letter to Dr. Mulloy, medical officer at the Blood Hospital. In his letter, Dr. Stone noted that the nuns had proven how effective this practice could be at aiding the hospital's success.[101] Allowing people to remain with family members encouraged reserve residents to remain in the hospital; it also fostered good relations with the community.

Nurses and nursing sisters used the different and often competing levels of authority to influence decisions within the hospital and decisions pertaining to medical matters at the reserve. At the Blood Hospital, the sisters found it helpful when one of the priests was present during an inspection.[102] There was strong animosity between the Anglican and Catholic missions at the Blood Reserve, mainly over the funding the Catholic hospital received from the federal government. To undermine the DIA's confidence in the nursing sisters, the Anglicans made it a point to regularly inspect the hospital and report on any real or imagined misdeeds.

The nursing sisters used the order's hierarchy not only to garner more authority but also to protect individual sisters from censure. Complaints from medical officers and DIA officials had to go through the proper channels: from the sister superior of the hospital to the superior general at Nicolet, the mother house in Edmonton. Sister St. Boissé, who had worked at the Blood Hospital since 1894, had a reputation for ignoring the medical officer's orders.[103] In the 1920s Dr. Kennedy complained first to the sister superior and then to the superior general and requested the immediate removal of Sister St. Boissé. The doctor believed that the sister had worked in the hospital far too long and was too set in her ways. Sister St. Boissé was, however, well liked by reserve residents and was not dismissed from the hospital. Instead she was transferred from the men's ward to the dispensary, where most of the work was carried out by female health workers.[104] The congregation's hierarchy also allowed nursing sisters an opportunity to address concerns about working conditions in the hospital. For example, in 1928 they complained to the reverend general about their lack of access to a priest and the sacrament of confession. They also felt that they were not at liberty to contact their superiors and that Sister St. Robitaille, the sister superior at their hospital, was at times an overly demanding taskmaster, especially with regard to the younger sisters.[105] In 1928 the reverend general admonished Sister St. Robitaille for treating her nursing sisters too harshly.[106] This incident shows that priorities changed depending on who was in charge. Under Sister St. Robitaille, patient care took precedence over the sisters' spiritual reflection – which was not always the case.

At posts where nurses were without other female support, they sought out the help of the only other health care worker at the reserve, the male doctor. Trained nurses in particular could appeal to the professional identity they shared with doctors. Miss Skuce, the public health nurse at the Sarcee Reserve, turned to Dr. Follett in 1915 when it became clear that she was expected to perform tasks she did not regard as an acceptable part of her job. In a letter to Rev. Tims, Dr. Follett outlined what he believed were Miss Skuce's responsibilities with regard to her work and living space: "Appointment of a trained nurse, who could do all dressings, keep charts daily for all patients, see any Indians at the reserve, give first aid in case of accident and give me some idea as to what any of them are suffering from, and let me know so that I can prepare intelligently the proper treatment before I make my visit."[107]

According to Dr. Follett, Miss Skuce was responsible for ensuring that her work space was clean following any medical procedures; however, scrubbing floors at the school was not part of her duties.[108] Dr. Follett's intervention did not resolve the situation, and Miss Skuce resigned little more than a month later. Conflicts like these often interfered with the ability of missions and the DIA to retain properly trained and conscientious health workers.

Miss Skuce's close association with the Sarcee Residential School complicated her job. Rev. Tims's expectations for female health care workers at residential schools were not unusual, just slightly dated. Given the broad range of nursing skills and training possessed by women in the nineteenth century, it was not unusual for a nurse to perform the duties of a servant, housekeeper, and nanny in addition to her therapeutic work. Women graduating from nursing programs at the turn of the century were, however, eager to separate themselves from the domestic work of nineteenth-century nursing practice. When the CMS hired Miss Bella to work as a nurse at the Sarcee Residential School in 1897, it was not unreasonable for Rev. Tims, the principal, to insist that Rutherford know how to cook, do needlework, and perform mission work.[109]

Transcultural Nursing?

Nursing scholarship in the United States offers valuable insight into the place, experience, work, and relationships of nurses in Aboriginal communities. Mary Ann Ruffing-Rahal's work on the public health nurse Elizabeth Forster looks at Forster's clinical practice among the Navajo during the early 1930s as an early example of transcultural nursing. Transcultural nursing involves using cultural knowledge in creative and meaningful ways to provide appropriate and beneficial care to members of diverse cultures. Nurses combine the cultural practices of their clients with their own nursing knowledge.[110] Although transcultural nursing was not officially identified in the United States until 1967, Ruffing-Rahal contends that public health nurses were building cross-cultural relationships with their clients in the United States as early as the 1880s.[111] Forster's personal letters reveal a health care provider who was sensitive to the cultural needs of her patients.[112] Although Ruffing-Rahal's study of Forster is uncritical and focuses on an exceptional nurse, Forster's case does highlight the importance of trying whenever possible to incorporate the experiences of individuals into an analysis of women's roles.

Emily Abel and Nancy Reifel offer another perspective on nurses' work in Aboriginal communities. Their work explores sets of skills and services that public health nurses made available to the Sioux, and they evaluate Aboriginal people's responses to these Euro-American women. They argue that the Sioux viewed nurses as "resources to be strategically and selectively used" and that they incorporated nurses' expertise into already existing Aboriginal models of healing.[113] Reifel contends that the work of public health nurses was easier for the Sioux to integrate into local curative practices because the skills public health nurses offered were more recognizable than the unfamiliar, brisk, and impersonal work of biomedical doctors.[114] Similar arguments have been made regarding the reaction of poor whites to biomedical practitioners in Natal, South Africa.[115]

Studies such as these are extremely valuable and suggest that there are many ways to examine sources. It is vital to consider the individual experiences of Euro-Canadian women. Yet we must not forget to place these women in a broader context, one that includes their participation (however tacit) in a system of health care intended to replace Aboriginal people's knowledge as well as their faith in that knowledge. Kate McPherson acknowledges the cultural complexities of Euro-Canadian women's work on reserves. Nurses served as front-line health care workers in Aboriginal communities and in the process articulated the colonizing agenda of the IHS. By trying to teach Aboriginal women European ideas of domesticity and sanitation, nurses were complicit in a public health campaign that stigmatized Aboriginal women for failing to become like their Euro-Canadian urban counterparts.[116] Some nurses chose to collaborate with Aboriginal healers or to form personal relationships in the community, but this was a matter of individual discretion and not a result of any departmental directives.[117]

Euro-Canadian women possessed greater opportunities than doctors to provide a broader range of services to Aboriginal people. Between 1880 and 1915, physicians were hired to work part-time on reserves; this practice, however, only entailed monthly visits and the occasional emergency call. Female medical missionaries, nursing sisters, and graduate nurses lived on reserves among their patients. This intimacy allowed female health workers greater opportunities to provide important and necessary resour-

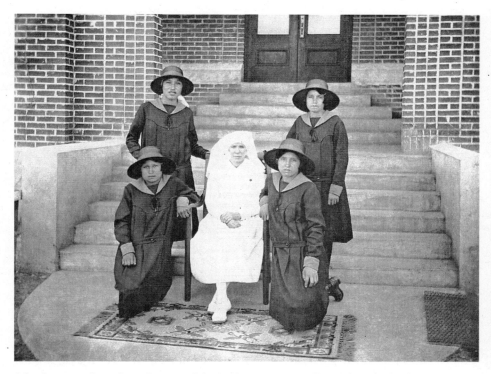

School nurse and pupils on the steps of the Anglican-run St. Paul's Residential School, Blood Reserve, 1927. *Back row, L-R:* Violet Creighton and Bella Healy. *Front row, L-R:* Jennie Healy, Miss Jane Megarry, and Olive Davis. | Courtesy Glenbow Archives NA-1811-35

ces to Aboriginal people. In some cases this led to close and significant relationships.

Many of the nuns, medical missionaries, matrons, and nurses tried to learn the language of their patients. Jane Megarry, who worked at the Blackfoot Hospital during the First World War, learned Blackfoot from a woman at the reserve and expressed joy at being able to communicate with her patients in their own language. Megarry commented that when "people were sick they preferred to speak in their own language because it was easier for them to describe how they felt and what they wanted."[118] Most of the nuns at the Blood Reserve likewise spoke Blackfoot – a skill the residents at the reserve found more useful to a greater number of people than English.[119] Besides learning to speak the language of their patients, some Euro-Canadian women made an effort to respect certain

Siksika customs. For example, family members were allowed to remain in the hospital with the patient to provide love and support. The Blackfoot Hospital provided room and board in exchange for odd jobs.[120] The Blood Hospital also allowed mothers to keep their children in the hospital with them.[121] Another example of cross-cultural nursing took place at the Blackfoot Hospital when Jane Megarry prepared the body of a patient following his death. In her diary she wrote: "I dressed the old man in all his splendid regalia as he had asked us to do. White buckskin coat and leggings – moccasins – all beaded with many colours of beautiful beads – and on his head the eagle feathered head dress."[122] Megarry went on to describe the mourning rituals observed by the man's family, some of which took place in the hospital.

It is possible that some skills provided by nurses and female health care workers were already familiar to Aboriginal people. Certain aspects of Western medicine might have been selectively incorporated into previously existing categories of medical knowledge in Aboriginal communities by the time these women arrived.[123] According to Reifel, public health nurses and the services they offered were judged by standards established for Aboriginal healers within their own communities. Evidence that this was the case at Treaty 7 reserves is extremely limited, but what is available suggests that some female health workers were accepted by members of the Aboriginal community. Miss Murray, the nurse at the Blackfoot Hospital in August 1910, was approached by an older man whom she had just treated. The man gave her several cans of fruit and vegetables that he had purchased specifically as payment for her healing services. On another occasion an outpatient attempted to pay Miss Murray a dollar for the treatment she had provided him.[124] She refused to accept these items as payment and only agreed to take them if they were considered donations to the hospital. Regardless, it is clear that her patients were offering a token payment for medical services rendered, much as they would have for any Aboriginal healer. In northwestern Plains societies a token or payment of gratitude to medicine men or healers was a widely accepted custom.[125]

There is also limited evidence that some nurses' strong character and dedication caused them to be much more effective in their dealings with Aboriginal people than other health care workers. These traits, according to Reifel, were highly valued among Aboriginal healers.[126] It is difficult to determine whether some Euro-Canadian women were more accepted than other health care personnel because the sources are Euro-Canadian and largely overlook the work of Euro-Canadian women. Megarry's reminiscences indicate that she felt as if she were part of the community – that she had formed friendships with local women, was invited to social gatherings, and was given an Aboriginal name by one of the chiefs at the Blackfoot Reserve.[127]

Another method for gauging the acceptance of Euro-Canadian women on reserves involves examining the complaints Aboriginal people levelled against Western health care workers. Aboriginal people were not shy about expressing their distrust of certain medical personnel. Doctors often earned the enmity of reserve residents. DIA records frequently refer to the need to remove certain doctors because of bad feelings toward them at a reserve.[128] This animosity often arose because a doctor had neglected his duties or had not responded promptly – or at all – to emergency calls. For good reason, a medical officer's failure to visit sick or dying residents created a great deal of bitterness and distrust among Aboriginal people. This was the case in 1912, when a young Siksika boy died without being treated by Dr. Rose. Rose had been notified by the boy's parents and Rev. Gibbon Stocken, the Anglican missionary at the Blackfoot Reserve, but he had failed to examine the boy.[129] Stocken wrote angrily to Indian agent J.H. Gooderham that oversights such as these on the part of the department's medical officer had led the Blackfoot to believe that the government did not care whether they lived or died.[130] The disregard of Western medical practitioners also ensured that Aboriginal peoples not only wanted to but also had to continue to rely on their own healers.

Even in cases where the doctor did respond to emergencies, Aboriginal people often regretted having called him because he arrived in a terrible mood. At the Blood Reserve, Dr. Edwards was notorious for arriving in bad temper and for treating patients "very roughly and perfunctory upon examination."[131] In a letter to the DIA, Indian agent W.J. Dilworth related an incident that he felt exemplified the drawbacks associated with employing Edwards as a medical officer: "The great reason why the doctor has lost the confidence of the Indians is ... the case of Tom Eagle Child's wife who had a sore leg. He pooh-poohed the idea of her having made much of the matter, but on her getting no better her husband took her to Lethbridge to Dr. Mewburn who found the bone diseased and who in their presence expressed his indignation at the neglect and fixed her up in a short time so she is perfectly well. This case is often mentioned to me."[132]

A similar situation prevailed at the Peigan Reserve. When asked to give his opinion regarding the reluctance of the Piikani to use the services provided by DIA medical officers, the Indian agent responded: "[The doctor] must possess the confidence of the Indian, and in order to obtain that confidence he must know them, not through the medium of periodical perfunctory visits to the reserve or emergency calls in isolated cases, but by being a member of the community, by being present at every sick bed, and prescribing for all ailments, great and small."[133]

It is not surprising, then, that Aboriginal people often went out of their way to avoid DIA medical officers. Sometimes, as was the case with Dr. Edwards, Indian agents echoed the criticisms made by reserve residents. But more often than not, Aboriginal people and their supposed ignorance of and prejudice against Western medicine were blamed, rather than the quality of care.[134]

It was physicians who received most of the attention for the health work performed on Treaty 7 reserves. Moreover, they took centre stage when complaints were made about inadequate medical services. Even so, female health care workers were not entirely immune from criticism. For instance, at one point – albeit in a later period – Dr. Alan Kennedy wrote to the superior general of the Sisters of Charity to request the removal of one of the sisters from the Blood Hospital. Kennedy did not question Sister St. Couture's nursing abilities; indeed, he believed she was a good nurse. The Kainai, however, did not like or trust her, and Kennedy believed it would be better for all if Couture worked among white people.[135]

Trustworthiness and strong character are essential to health workers and caregivers in any community. Some health care workers formed lasting friendships with Aboriginal people; others clearly did not. The growing institutionalization of DIA facilities in the early twentieth century would fundamentally alter the relationships that white caregivers and Aboriginal patients had developed up to that point.

Conclusion

The financial relationship that developed between the federal state and the churches facilitated the establishment of a Western health care regime on reserves in southern Alberta. Catholic orders and congregations and Protestant missionary organizations, concerned about the poor health of their Treaty 7 congregations and wanting to extend their reach into communities, expanded their health work by founding hospitals, dispensaries, and school infirmaries and by pressing the DIA to fund these new initiatives. The less expensive labour of female missionaries, some of whom possessed formal nursing training, was essential to the development of this system. Few historical works have focused specifically on the role that female health care workers played in delivering Western curative services to Aboriginal peoples. Historians who have examined the effects of Western medicine on Aboriginal peoples in Canada have failed to differentiate between the medical work of Euro-Canadian women and that of men. As a result, the prevailing image of government-run health care on reserves is that it was undertaken mainly by male physicians.

Female nursing attendants on reserves were in a difficult spot. They were already considered less than equal because of their profession and their gender. Furthermore, they were subject to multiple levels of authority on reserves: they had to contend with DIA officials, church officials, medical officers, and matrons and hospital administrators. In urban hospitals, graduate nurses and nurses in training could rely on other nurses for support and advice, whereas on reserves they often worked alone. Reserve hospitals were understaffed, and nurses among the Nakoda and Tsuu T'ina generally worked alone. In contrast, the Grey Nuns at the Blood Hospital had a community of women to turn to when faced with difficult situations and when conflicts had to be negotiated between the nuns and the department, the Indian agent, or the medical officer. Finally, in the absence of doctors, nurses and female nursing attendants were often left to make difficult medical decisions and to perform procedures that did not normally fall within nursing practice.

Euro-Canadian women also developed extremely complicated relationships with Aboriginal people. As purveyors of Western medicine and nursing care, it was possible for them to improve the lives of Aboriginal people. Advances in treatments and aseptic techniques at the turn of the last century presented improvements in Western medicine and medical care. These advances were tempered, however, by the intersection of medicine and colonialism. The provision of medical services by the churches and the state was not entirely about addressing ill health in Aboriginal communities. Western medicine was accompanied by a host of cultural and social implications. The work of churches was always informed by their members' commitment to Christian conversion; the efforts of the state were intimately connected to nation building and assimilation. As the DIA became more directly involved in Western health services in Treaty 7 communities, greater emphasis was placed on *where* Western medicine was practised and on the skill sets and training of female health workers. In addition, public health rather than religion came to inform the relations that Euro-Canadian women developed with Aboriginal communities, especially women and children. All the while, mission organizations and their female workers continued their involvement – if somewhat more circumspectly – in Treaty 7 communities, fighting the DIA for dwindling resources. Stronger DIA management meant increasingly limited health care options for Aboriginal peoples.

6

Taking over the System

Graduate Nurses, Nursing Sisters, Female Attendants, and Indian Health Services, 1915-30

After 1915 the Department of Indian Affairs (DIA) began to take over the administration of health services from the churches. Instead of rebuilding rundown and obsolescent church facilities, the DIA simply took over existing hospitals, school infirmaries, and dispensaries. Western health services therefore changed very little during this period; indeed, an informal relationship often persisted between the churches and the government. When it could, the DIA continued to use female missionaries as health care workers because they were affordable and available, in addition to being committed to the state's civilizing agenda. In sum, the withdrawal of the churches and their personnel was an uneven process. Laywomen did not outnumber women with religious affiliations at DIA institutions until the 1920s. Nurses played important roles in the DIA apparatus, and the performance of gender in state-run health care regimes shaped the character of nursing and educational services.

Throughout this period of transition, Euro-Canadian women remained the front-line health care workers in the Treaty 7 area. It was they who carried out most of the medical and nursing care in DIA institutions. Many of the caring duties that Euro-Canadian women performed in DIA hospitals remained the same as those carried out earlier by missionaries; however, women working for the DIA were expected to possess a different set of professional skills. In the late 1920s, the DIA intensified its effort to employ nurses with formal training, and female mission workers were not exempted from this policy. The ability to assist doctors and carry out complex procedures became an ever more important prerequisite for female

DIA health care workers, as well as a point of contestation in reserve facilities, where female mission workers with years of practical experience and knowledge as healers and caregivers were being pushed aside to make room for inexperienced women with formal training. And even while expectations regarding nursing qualifications were being debated, female health workers had to navigate ever more complicated relationships with Indian agents, local doctors, the DIA, and church authorities. Hospitals in urban areas had a recognized chain of command and established protocols. The situation was much more complex for female health workers on reserves, who often worked on their own and were forced to make difficult decisions. As female workers and employees of the state, they faced dual restraints on their autonomy and in the relationships they formed with Aboriginal women and the reserve community.[1]

The public health work that female workers carried out, rather than religion, became the cornerstone of DIA health policy. The DIA believed that instruction in sanitation and hygiene was the solution to the ill health and poor living conditions faced by many Aboriginal peoples. As a consequence, the DIA did not replace mission medical personnel when they were withdrawn, even though conditions remained poor. Instead, it launched a system of public health and travelling nurses whose principal task was to instruct Aboriginal women in Euro–Canadian-style domesticity and child care. This educational work soon became the cornerstone of Euro-Canadian women's health work on Treaty 7 reserves. Many of these workers, unlike their missionary counterparts, were not stationed permanently on reserves. They often arrived during medical emergencies and left soon afterwards, much like DIA medical officers. These modifications to the work and place of female health care workers in Treaty 7 communities fundamentally altered the relationship between Western health practitioners and Aboriginal peoples, for they introduced a new patient-practitioner relationship.

The DIA Health Care Regime

The federal government had contributed personnel and financial support to the mission-based hospitals, school infirmaries, and dispensaries since the 1890s. In 1915 the DIA moved to directly control health care services on Treaty 7 reserves. In part the DIA was responding to the withdrawal of mission organizations from the home field. For instance, the Methodist Church closed the Morley Residential School and its hospital in 1911 and ceased to have a significant educational or medical presence at the Stoney Reserve.² But the DIA primarily assumed direct control over Treaty 7 health services because of escalating medical costs, the continued influence of Aboriginal healers, and persisting ill health in reserve communities.

During his time as chief accountant and superintendent of Indian education, Duncan Campbell Scott had been dismayed by the escalating costs of providing medical services to Aboriginal peoples.³ In 1913, soon after his appointment as deputy superintendent of Indian affairs, Scott curbed departmental spending by adopting a more active role in the administration and supervision of medical services for Aboriginal peoples. Of particular concern was Aboriginal people's use of off-reserve doctors and medical facilities. Beginning during the fur trade era and extending into the twentieth century, Aboriginal peoples in the Treaty 7 area had selectively sought out European medicine on their own terms. With the growth of white settlement and the availability of physicians and hospitals, they continued to rely on non-Aboriginal medicine and visited local doctors and nearby hospitals for treatment. Aboriginal people based their medical choices on the quality and effectiveness of treatment and on the perceived origins and nature of disease, which meant that they often sought out the help of non-DIA physicians to acquire better medical care or a second opinion.

Aboriginal people's resort to Western medicine was not entirely a matter of medical pluralism. They were using services and resources that they believed had been promised by treaty. Their insistence on using off-reserve health care facilities, despite mounting DIA condemnation, reveals that they understood health care as a treaty right. This practice was also a comment on the state of DIA health services more generally. Indeed, the healing and caregiving choices made by Aboriginal people during these years were much more complicated than DIA records reveal. The therapeutic system that developed in the twentieth century in the Treaty 7 area included Aboriginal *and* European medical practices and beliefs.⁴ The texts of anthropologists who observed Aboriginal people in southern Alberta during the 1930s and interviews conducted with Aboriginal elders point to a more complex and pluralistic pattern of healing and caregiving.⁵

The strategies employed by Treaty 7 peoples to obtain the best possible medical treatment frustrated the DIA, especially given that Aboriginal people were reluctant to use the department's own facilities. When Scott asked Dr. Steele in 1918 why the Kainai were not using the hospital, Steele replied that the hospital faced a "deplorable lack of modern conveniences."⁶ Instead of acknowledging the truth of these statements, Indian agents labelled Aboriginal people as ungrateful and undeserving. The DIA tried to limit the medical treatment and nursing-care options available to Aboriginal people at off-reserve facilities. To encourage attendance at reserve institutions, the DIA refused to pay for treatment at Euro-Canadian hospitals except in exceptional circumstances. It also turned down requests for passes and made the character of individuals relevant when deciding who did and who did not deserve medical treatment.[7]

Indian agent W. Pocklington wrote a letter to the department in 1890 in which he admitted that he had often given passes to Kainai people who were sick and who wanted to visit a doctor in Lethbridge or Fort Macleod.[8] He assured the department, however, that these requests had been granted only after a thorough inquiry into the individual's character to determine that a visit to the doctor was legitimate. Pocklington's letter offers no details as to who was responsible for paying the doctor's bills. Physicians throughout southern Alberta often approached the DIA for reimbursement for the treatments they had provided to Aboriginal people. For example, Dr. J.H. Rivers of Raymond, Alberta, requested compensation from the department for medical services rendered to the child of a Kainai man who had been working for a local rancher and who had left without paying. Rivers' application was denied.[9] This was not an isolated episode. The DIA's refusal to pay medical bills undermined the willingness of non-department physicians and hospitals to provide treatment to Aboriginal people. It also limited Aboriginal people's therapeutic options.

When Aboriginal people did not trust the diagnosis or treatment provided by a DIA physician, they looked elsewhere. Depending on the illness, one option was to approach an Aboriginal healer. Another was to seek out a second medical opinion. In 1905 a Kainai band chief who was dissatisfied with the results of Dr. O.C. Edwards' examination determined that with or without the DIA's permission, he would go to Calgary and see an eye specialist. The chief intended to pay for the treatment himself.[10] The department's decision in this matter was not recorded. In other situations, Aboriginal people were willing to pay for medical treatment that the department would not. Dr. James Lafferty, a DIA medical officer, wrote to Agent Wilson in 1901 to ask for permission to operate on an Aboriginal man with scrofula who had come to his office in Calgary accompanied by Father Davis.[11] The patient had paid for both train fares and was determined to obtain treatment from Lafferty. He most likely would have been turned down for treatment by the DIA's reserve hospital, and he had brought Father Davis with him to add weight to his request and ensure its approval. It is not known whether the request was approved. The point is that the presence of Father Davis shows that the man was very much aware of the politics of accessing health care.

The second factor that propelled the DIA to take an active supervisory role in health services was the resilience of Aboriginal healing practices. The DIA held Aboriginal doctors responsible for the general failure of Euro-Canadian health care professionals and institutions that the government provided. Western medicine's failure to make serious inroads into Aboriginal communities was blamed on the "older and more traditional" elements of reserve communities. The department contended that senior band members and male Aboriginal healers were using their influence and authority to discourage people from attending DIA hospitals and following the instructions of department medical staff.[12]

Aboriginal people turned to healers and caregivers depending on their needs, and they based their medical decisions on the proven effectiveness of particular treatments. Thus, when Aboriginal medicine or allopathy failed, people pursued an alternative course of treatment. The state understood medicine and medical practice in black-and-white terms: Western medicine and science embodied the superiority of Euro-Canadian society, whereas Aboriginal medicine exemplified Aboriginal people's backwardness.

Anthropologists Lucien and Jane Richardson Hanks interviewed Aboriginal people in the Treaty 7 area during the late 1930s. They found that Aboriginal health care practices were still being used among the Blackfoot and that "specialists for swellings, blood poisoning, female complaints etc., nearly every cluster of houses can produce at least one such practitioner."[13] When DIA institutions failed to meet people's medical and caregiving needs, there were well-known individuals in the community who could. For instance, a healer named Crooked Meat Strings provided medical care for Tony Crane Bear when he was kicked in the head by a horse, which left him suffering constant headaches and seizures.[14] After an unsuccessful visit to a white doctor, Tony Crane Bear was left on his own to deal with his illness.[15] Crooked Meat Strings treated him, making him drink from the bark of chokecherries every day as treatment for the headaches.[16] Mary White Elk also related a story about her son's treatment at the Blood Hospital. When it became clear that no one was going to be able to cure his illness, she stepped in and did so herself.[17]

More recent accounts highlight the persistence of Aboriginal healing practices. During a 1983 interview, Kainai elder Rufus Goodstriker shared an episode from his childhood. As a young man, Goodstriker had died and was revived with mouth-to-mouth resuscitation by a medicine woman.[18]

Later, when he was diagnosed with gallstones, he visited a medicine woman who gave him some sort of mixture to drink and prayed for him.[19] Goodstriker was cured of his gallstones and did not need surgery. Annie Bare Shin Bone likewise recounted that when she had fallen very ill as a child, her grandmother had rubbed her body with medicine and prayed. This ritual was repeated several times until Annie recovered.[20] Another example comes from Mike Mountain Horse's semi-autobiographical work *My People the Bloods,* in which Mountain Horse describes several instances in which he observed the work of medicine men and was himself treated for rheumatism.[21] Finally, Joan Scott-Brown, in her 1977 study on Nakoda ethnobotany, found that the Nakoda community had used the local health clinic at the reserve, but if the doctor's cures were unsatisfactory or slow in taking effect, or if the illness was a chronic condition, the Nakoda had sought out the services of a medicine woman.[22]

The failure of Western medicine to replace Aboriginal practices led DIA employees like Indian agent W.J. Dilworth at the Blood Reserve to blame the persistence of medicine men on the department's indulgence of Aboriginal people. He complained that because "[we have] cater[ed] to much to his desires ... little if any actual progress has been made, Indian doctors and superstitions are still paramount."[23] He believed that Aboriginal people should be compelled to get medical treatment and went so far as to recommend that a system of mandatory medical treatment, similar to the one used in the British army, be instituted on reserves.[24] The failure of hospitals, nurses, and doctors to produce the desired results was not blamed on a chronically underfunded health care system but rather on the older and less assimilated members of the community.[25]

The final factor that influenced the shape of DIA health services was the prevalence of infectious diseases in Treaty 7 communities. Scott believed that, given the pervasiveness of certain diseases despite the presence of Western medical care, more money spent on hospitals and medical treatments would not solve the problem of ill health in Aboriginal communities. By 1915, DIA officials had declared tuberculosis to be an endemic disease on most Aboriginal reserves. Indian commissioner William Morris Graham wrote to Indian agent Tom Graham of the Peigen Reserve in 1922 that "scrofula and other kindred ailments, these are found to exist on all reserves to a greater or lesser extent."[26] Graham believed that the department's resources would be better spent educating Aboriginal people about "the value of fresh air, the necessity of proper food, keeping their persons and houses clean, and the observation of the laws of sanitation."[27] Disease and ill health would be dealt with through appropriate training and knowledge and, in this context, Western modes of housekeeping and child care took on new meaning and importance.

The department was prepared to use all means at its disposal to ensure that Aboriginal people adhered to the training and advice DIA employees had to offer. To ensure that Aboriginal people embraced what they believed were modern practices of hygiene and sanitation, DIA officials began to implement more coercive measures. An amendment to the Indian Act passed in 1914 gave the department full responsibility for maintaining proper sanitary conditions on reserves and in all departmental institutions. The same amendment empowered the superintendent general of Indian affairs to develop and enforce sanitary regulations for the prevention of disease and for the maintenance of streets, houses, and public buildings.[28] It also allowed for the forcible medical treatment of Aboriginal people. Reserve residents who did not comply with physicians' orders were removed from the community and sent to off-reserve facilities for an undetermined time. A person who refused to submit to a doctor's examination or treatment could be punished by a fine or imprisonment. Under the guise of public health and disease prevention, DIA employees measured the danger posed by reserve residents – especially women – according to the degree to which Aboriginal people subscribed to Euro-Canadian conventions regarding therapeutic practices, personal dress, nutrition, housekeeping, and child care.[29] The 1914 amendment therefore gave the department the power to enforce policies, and it subjected domestic space to greater scrutiny by using the language of science and contagion to justify interference by the state and its agents.

In its quest for fiscal restraint, the DIA bureaucracy actually grew during these years. Efforts to reduce medical costs were accompanied in the 1920s by the centralization of medical services for Aboriginal peoples within the DIA bureaucracy. When Dr. Peter Bryce was fired in 1913 as chief medical officer, the position remained vacant until the appointment of Dr. E.L. Stone in 1927. After 1921, medical services were managed by the department's accountant, who was less than sympathetic or generous. The health needs of Aboriginal people continued to be a low priority for the DIA and for the federal government more generally. In 1919, when the Department of Health was created, Parliament did not include medical services for Aboriginal peoples within this new department. Not until 1927 did the DIA establish a Medical Branch to administer the health needs of Aboriginal peoples. Medical historian T. Kue Young contends that the primary reason for formally creating Indian Health Services (IHS) in 1927 was to monitor medical costs more closely.[30]

Before being appointed as the DIA's chief medical superintendent, Dr. Stone had worked as a physician for the department for several years. In his new post, he carried out the policies that Scott had put in place over the previous decade. Fiscal constraint and responsibility therefore remained the DIA's governing principles.[31] Prior to his appointment, Stone had been responsible for visiting agencies to treat patients and perform health surveys. In 1926 he had been placed in charge of the DIA hospital at Norway House, Manitoba. Like his medical contemporaries, he recognized that tuberculosis was a problem in Aboriginal communities, yet he did not see the improvement of Aboriginal peoples' standard of living as the solution. Like his counterparts in urban public health agencies, he believed that instruction in sanitation and hygiene was a more important tool for combatting disease than improved material conditions and access to long-term treatment.[32]

A transformation in the living standards of all Aboriginal peoples in southern Alberta would have required a financial commitment that the federal government was unwilling to make. Instead, it instituted a program of field matrons – and, after 1922, travelling public health nurses – to instruct Aboriginal women in the proper precepts of home and child care. Most field matrons were either the wives of local ranchers or female missionaries hired by the DIA to instruct Aboriginal women in the domestic arts. Field matrons organized mothers' meetings and held classes in knitting, sewing, and cooking. Even though they did not possess any medical training, the field matrons were supplied with drugs, dressings, and simple remedies and expected in the absence of trained medical personnel to deal with all medical emergencies. In 1927 there were only five field matrons working in Manitoba, Alberta, and Saskatchewan.[33]

The field matron program in Canada paralleled developments in the United States. According to Lisa Emmerich, "the field matron program owed its existence to the belief that the power of domesticity could bring Native Americans closer to the goal of assimilation."[34] Upon working in reserve communities, however, field matrons quickly altered their work to fit the needs of Treaty 7 peoples. Health care consequently became a regular component of their routines.[35] The position of field matron was indicative of the department's commitment to cost cutting. Instead of hiring trained health professionals, the DIA employed local, untrained Euro-Canadian women and paid them less. Aboriginal people were aware that these women lacked training and often sought treatment in off-reserve facilities.

The program of travelling public health nurses was launched in 1922 to extend the existing educational and public health work of missionaries and field matrons. The work of travelling and public health nurses blended curative and nursing care with instruction on domestic hygiene and child care. Travelling nurses were in charge of a single district, and one nurse was responsible for all of the reserves in southern Alberta. Only four nurses administered the three Prairie provinces.[36] In areas where the department regarded the Aboriginal population as too insignificant to justify the expense of a public health nurse, the services of a Euro-Canadian woman without formal nursing training (i.e., a field matron) was retained.[37]

During the 1920s, ill health underscored by high infant-mortality rates continued to be a concern in Aboriginal communities. Around this time the DIA took over existing reserve hospitals.[38] By the late 1920s, department officials were attempting to ensure that all IHS services were provided in a hospital environment under the supervision of appropriate medical personnel. Nurses continued to visit people in their homes, but physicians were expected to carry out their work in the hospital or school infirmary. The DIA built hospitals on every reserve in the Treaty 7 area as a means to transfer medical treatment and nursing care from informal settings to hospitals and institutional spaces. The growth of DIA hospitals reflected the changing place of hospitals in Euro-Canadian society. The late nineteenth and early twentieth centuries witnessed the shift from charity hospitals as places in which only the poor and destitute received treatment to scientific medical facilities in which people expected that they would be cured.[39] The dormitory-style wards that continued to be used in reserve hospitals were similar to the large public wards used by working-class patients in urban centres. By this time more and more white middle-class patients were demanding access to private or semi-private rooms.[40]

In 1923 the DIA took over management of the Blackfoot Hospital from the Anglican Church and used band funds to rebuild the facility.[41] The new building had two storeys and thirty-five beds and was staffed by lay nurses.[42] The DIA took over administration of the Blood Hospital in 1928, expanded it, and moved it from Standoff to Cardston. The Grey Nuns, however, continued to work in the Blood Hospital until 1954. During the late 1920s and 1930s, the DIA built hospitals at the Sarcee, Stoney, and Peigan reserves.[43] In 1921, under the direction of Dr. Thomas Murray, newly appointed Indian agent for the Sarcee Reserve, the Sarcee Residential School was converted into a tuberculosis sanatorium for the twenty-nine students who attended it.[44] The staff comprised a practical nurse, a cook,

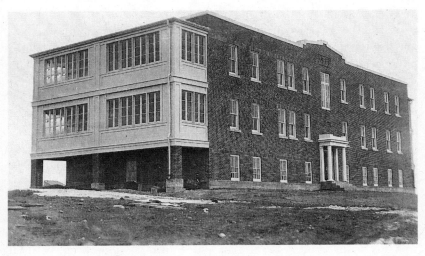

The newly renovated Blood Hospital at Cardston, Alberta, 1929. | Courtesy Grey Nuns Archives, Montreal

and a schoolteacher. A hospital was built at the Peigan Reserve in 1927, and it housed eight beds, one graduate nurse, and a housekeeper. The hospital at Morley was built in 1935 and opened in January 1936 with ten beds and a staff of two graduate nurses.[45]

Dr. Harold McGill was appointed deputy superintendent general of Indian affairs in 1932. McGill's appointment had little impact on the IHS's operations, however. McGill had first come to Calgary in 1910 and had served as a medical officer for the Tsuu T'ina before enlisting in the army during the First World War. On his return from Europe, he resumed his post with the DIA.[46] Under McGill the IHS grew very slowly. By 1935 the DIA's Medical Branch employed eleven full-time medical officers, eight Indian agents who had medical training, and 250 physicians available on a part-time or on-call basis.[47] A grand total of eleven field nurses were engaged by the branch. In 1934 the average yearly cost of medical treatment for a Euro-Canadian was $31.00; the average cost for an Aboriginal person was $9.60.[48]

Health care services for Aboriginal people would remain a low priority for the federal government until after the Second World War. In 1936 the DIA – including its Medical Branch – would be absorbed by the Department of Mines and Natural Resources. This reorganization reflected the Great Depression's impact on government resources and the minor importance assigned to Aboriginal issues in general.[49]

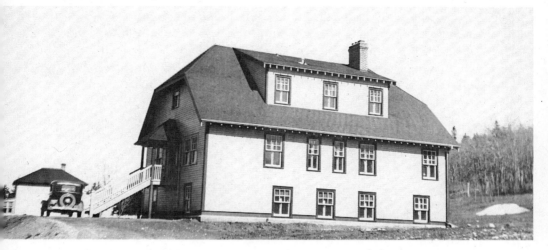

The newly built DIA hospital at Morley, 1935. | Courtesy Glenbow Archives PD-338-42

The Place of Nurses within DIA Health Services

After the First World War, securing high-quality medical personnel remained a problem for DIA officials. Physicians continued to be hired on a part-time basis, and they visited reserves once a week and were on-call for emergencies. The Blackfoot Hospital was visited weekly by Dr. Rose, who later became the medical officer for the entire reserve. Dr. Edwards was the medical officer for the Kainai and the Piikani between 1901 and 1915. He lived near the agency in Cardston and travelled once a week to the Blood Hospital, the Anglican mission school, and the Peigan Reserve. The Kainai community's dislike of Edwards did not prevent community members from visiting his wife, the well-known maternal feminist Henrietta Muir Edwards. She was often visited by reserve residents "seeking medicine from the dispensary, food, and conversation."[50] Her grandchildren remembered that she "kept a pot of soup on the stove, never locked the door, welcomed many visitors, and fed everyone."[51] Edwards died at the beginning of the First World War, and the shortage of doctors following the outbreak of hostilities made it much more difficult for the department to find good physicians.

Confronted with ongoing shortages of competent medical doctors, the DIA – much like the churches and their mission societies – continued to rely on the more affordable labour of female health workers. Euro-Canadian women who worked as graduate and public health nurses, nursing sisters, and nursing attendants remained an integral part of the health system after the DIA took over its management. Euro-Canadian women were full-time employees in hospitals, school infirmaries, and dispensaries. They also served as temporary emergency health care workers and as travelling public health nurses.

The new hospitals at the Sarcee, Stoney, and Peigan reserves, like the ones at the Blackfoot and Blood reserves, were run mainly by women, supplemented by the part-time services of a doctor. After 1923 only the Blood Hospital continued to be staffed by a female religious congregation. After 1928 the facility was staffed by three nuns who were graduate nurses and by several nursing sisters with a great deal of experience though no formal training. By centralizing medical care on reserves, the DIA hoped to reduce medical costs while maintaining a certain level of care.[52] But centralization also altered the relationship between practitioners and patients and limited the treatment options available to Aboriginal people.

Department officials believed that once Aboriginal people adopted an appropriate Euro-Canadian lifestyle, their health problems would be resolved. According to Scott, education offered a less costly and more lasting solution to Aboriginal people's health problems. The DIA's policies and its staff and resource allocations between 1915 and 1930 period reflected this focus.

The DIA directed its resources toward instructing Aboriginal people in hygiene and sanitation. One result was that when a health crisis arose, the department's response was slow, temporary, and inadequate. Throughout the late nineteenth and early twentieth centuries, DIA medical officers regularly quarantined reserves, DIA hospitals, and residential schools during outbreaks of smallpox, diphtheria, measles, whooping cough, and influenza. On reserves without a DIA hospital, graduate nurses were hired to handle medical emergencies and quarantines. Once the emergency had passed, nursing services were withdrawn. This was the case on August 5, 1916, when measles broke out at the Peigan Reserve. A nurse was stationed full-time near the Indian agent's house, and all patients were brought within walking distance of her quarters so that she could attend them.[53] The nurse left shortly before the outbreak ended.

A similar situation developed in 1919, when the hospital at the Blackfoot Reserve was quarantined during an outbreak of scarlet fever. A public health nurse, Le Drew, was brought in to set up a temporary hospital. The medical officer for the reserve was quarantined as well. Le Drew took over responsibility for supervising the students at the school, visiting the homes in which scarlet fever was reported, and running a dispensary out of the Indian agent's office every day from 11:00 a.m. to 12:30 p.m.[54] After the emergency was believed to have passed, she was assigned elsewhere. Temporary postings made it inevitable that the relationships nurses formed with their patients differed from the ones medical missionaries had developed.

Even though tuberculosis is highly infectious, no steps were taken on Treaty 7 reserves to immediately quarantine people infected with it. Children remained in schools among their peers, and reserve residents rarely used the hospital. According to historian Maureen Lux, in spite of the pervasiveness of respiratory infections, they were only the third most common reason for visiting the dispensary at the Blood Hospital. This was the case even in 1906-07, when Dr. Bryce submitted a report that attributed half the deaths at the Blood Reserve to TB.[55] The lack of interest that reserve residents showed in using reserve hospitals had several bases. Dr. Edwards, the physician for the Blood Hospital, "treated most respiratory complaints with a mixture of expectorant and demulcent herbs and aromatics."[56] Such therapeutics mirrored many Aboriginal remedies for respiratory problems – remedies that included sweat lodges, infusions of yellow berries, and tea made from willow bark.[57] If residents could readily obtain such treatments elsewhere, why attend the reserve hospital?

But the second and most significant deterrent to inpatient care was that the treatment for TB often entailed a prolonged and isolating hospital stay. Few people were willing to submit themselves to a treatment that required them to abandon home and family for an indefinite time. For this reason, temporary facilities were often set up to treat the immediate and visible symptoms of TB. For example, a dressing station was set up near the Peigan Reserve in March 1922 on the advice of Dr. Gillespie, the DIA medical officer, and Miss Ramage, the public health nurse. Indian agent Tom Graham established the station so that outpatients could have their scrofulous sores washed and dressed daily by the nurse. (Scrofula is a glandular form of TB that affects the lymph nodes in the neck.) The DIA's permission to open this temporary nursing station was short-lived. Indian commissioner Graham withdrew his consent less than two months later. Graham did not see the utility of maintaining the dressing station, given what he believed to be the universal nature of TB on reserves. He instead advocated teaching Aboriginal people "correct living habits."[58] As early as 1905, DIA employees were linking improved home life to community well-being.[59] They had yet to link better living conditions and improved nutrition to better health. The responsibility of educating Aboriginal people fell to the public health nurses and field matrons employed by the department, all of whom were only sporadically present.

The situation remained critical for the Piikani, and in April the following year it was deemed necessary to set up another small infirmary to treat the same health problems. Indian agent Arthur described this facility as unsuitable because it was not furnished, had no running water, and consisted of only one room and a kitchen. All of the patients were kept together in the one room.[60] In spite of the temporary hospital's shortcomings, many people came for treatment, and the nurse performed at least sixteen dressings a day for patients suffering from scrofula and other TB-related illnesses. Reserve health care remained inconsistent and short-term, however. The episodic posting of nurses during health emergencies reflected the department's general policy on health care.

Persistent poor health in some communities meant that nurses could not be withdrawn. In communities where health conditions were considered especially poor, the DIA paid for a full-time nurse to remain at the reserve. The permanent posting of a nurse usually occurred after complaints had been made by non-Aboriginal people about health conditions or after high death rates among children were observed. In most cases the parents – especially mothers – were held responsible for these conditions. This was the case at the Sarcee Reserve in 1915 and among the Nakoda in 1927 and 1928. The DIA agreed to appoint a full-time graduate nurse for the Sarcee Reserve after the new medical officer, Dr. Follett, revealed shocking rates of TB infection among residential school students and reserve residents. In 1928 a nurse was posted at Morley after appallingly high rates of infant mortality were disclosed to the public by an unknown source within the department.

The DIA agreed to hire a nurse on the condition she make her services available both to students at the Sarcee Residential School and to reserve residents.[61] The DIA paid the nurse's salary, and the Anglican school provided room and board and space for a dispensary.[62] Rev. J.W. Tims, the school principal, was satisfied with this arrangement because the nurse was a member of the Church of England and conformed to all the rules and regulations of the mission. The department was happy with this arrangement because the contract saved the federal government five hundred dollars a year.[63] This example reminds us that the withdrawal of churches from the provision of health care was uneven: there were times when the female health care work of churches continued.[64]

In 1928, in similar circumstances, the DIA retained a full-time nurse's services for the Morley reserve after R.B. Bennett, leader of the federal

Conservative Party, complained to Scott, in March 1927, about high infant morality rates among the Nakoda. Unlike the Anglican Church, which maintained a presence in the Tsuu T'ina community, the Methodist Church was not involved in the provision of health services, having withdrawn any significant presence at that reserve following the closure of the McDougall Orphanage almost fifteen years earlier. Scott immediately authorized the hiring of a graduate nurse to address infant mortality. Believing that the Nakoda were unaware of health conditions on their reserve, Scott directed the nurse to inform the Nakoda about the gravity of their situation. She was also told to pay particular attention to expectant mothers and young children.[65] Her DIA salary was $960 a year. Her job description was as follows: "To conduct an intensive training campaign on the care of children with mothers and expectant mothers; to give special attention to infants and young children; to report to the agent when it is necessary to have the services of a doctor; to administer necessary medicines in cases of minor illnesses, and to have such care and treatment as a graduate nurse is called upon to administer."[66]

This position was formalized at Morley in 1928.[67] The permanent presence of a graduate nurse on a reserve was unique to the Tsuu T'ina and Nakoda: nurses were rarely stationed in one place permanently unless they worked at a DIA hospital. A nurse was usually retained only for as long as the DIA thought she was absolutely necessary. Temporary female health workers had no opportunity to develop relations with the community based on mutual trust and respect. Mothers remained reluctant to use the nurse's services and often hid their children when she came to visit. As a result, assumptions about the causes of ill health in Aboriginal communities were based on preconceived notions, which remained rooted in gendered assumptions about domesticity and the reluctance of Aboriginal women to conform to Euro-Canadian modes of child care. The inconsistent pattern regarding where and when nurses were placed in southern Alberta's Aboriginal communities reminds us that interactions with DIA health services in this region were an erratic patchwork.

Nursing Practice and Training

The work of DIA nurses was similar to the work carried out by the nurses and untrained female attendants employed by mission societies. The largest group to use reserve hospitals continued to be students and their families. Most of the nursing care undertaken by Euro-Canadian women both inside and outside hospitals involved people suffering from respiratory conditions, digestive tract problems, and ear, eye, and throat problems.[68] The dispensary at the hospital or school or near the Indian agent's office continued to be the place where most people sought treatment on reserves.

The kinds of illnesses that propelled Aboriginal people to seek treatment reflected poor living conditions in their communities and shaped the kinds of work that Euro-Canadian nurses performed. Lifestyle changes and improvements in living standards that were extending life expectancy and decreasing infant mortality among Euro-Canadians were not occurring at the same pace among Aboriginal peoples.[69] In 1918 a trust fund of $1 million was created when the Siksika reluctantly surrendered large tracts of land. The first thing the band council did was provide meals for everyone. It then petitioned the DIA to renovate the hospital.[70] That the Siksika did these things indicates that the basic needs of many people were not being met and that the community itself viewed health care and nutrition as priorities.

After 1915, Euro-Canadian women's educational roles expanded and greater importance was placed on prevention rather than medical care and treatment. Yet, despite the introduction of scientific medicine and germ theory, solutions to ill health and disease on reserves remained rooted in nineteenth-century ideas about race and culture. Officials with the DIA believed that it was futile to treat symptoms when the cause of disease was entrenched in Aboriginal culture. When Dr. J.J. Wall was hired by the DIA in the 1920s to study the prevalence of trachoma in western Canada, he characterized reserves as "wells of contagion" and used racial and cultural characteristics to explain the pervasiveness of trachoma among Aboriginal peoples.[71] In particular, he singled out older Aboriginal women's headscarves and love for their grandchildren as sources of infection. The care of children by elderly family members was regarded as a problem rather than as a solution or strategy to deal with pressing issues of child care. Nor did Wall's report address the urgent health care needs of many people in Treaty 7 communities.

Those female workers who were stationed permanently in Treaty 7 communities – especially Euro-Canadian women who worked outside institutional bounds – were exposed to a wider range of medical concerns and continued to perform a diverse range of curative services. The reports submitted by the nurses at the Sarcee Reserve describe a variety of medical situations that the nurses dealt with regularly. Agnes Huncomb's report recounts her activities for December 1916: monitoring the condition of schoolchildren suffering from TB, grippe, and adenitis; and at the reserve itself, attending a birth, vaccinating nineteen children, and treating a woman who had frozen her feet. Other nurses at the Sarcee Reserve described lancing abscesses as well as treating eye inflammations, burns, foot injuries, coughs and colds, dysentery, nicotine poisoning, outbreaks of chicken pox and measles, and rheumatism. They also made maternity visits. The nurses dispensed medicinals such as eye water, iodine, cough syrup, camphor oil, Epsom salts, castor oil, olive oil, and various ointments.[72] Nurses dealt with a multitude of health problems that ranged from illnesses associated with poverty and occupational injuries to normal life events such as childhood colds and pregnancy.

Doctors continued to rely on the judgment of nurses to assess the severity of medical cases. In 1917 Nurse Maude Hill diagnosed one of the children from the Sarcee Residential School with tubercular peritonitis and arranged for his immediate removal to a hospital in Calgary for surgery.[73] Dr. Follett, who was unable to travel to the reserve, agreed with Hill's assessment and helped her deal not only with the Indian agent but also with the principal of the Anglican residential school, Rev. Tims, who disagreed with Hill's decision. A similar incident occurred at the Blood Reserve in 1926, when Dr. Alan Kennedy, the reserve's medical attendant, refused to attend a woman suffering from postpartum complications at her home. Kennedy was persuaded only after Sister St. Robitaille examined the woman and decided she needed immediate medical attention.[74] Trusting her assessment, Kennedy agreed to treat the woman, but she died before the doctor arrived.[75] Kennedy had every faith in the nursing sisters at the Blood Hospital and relied on them to carry out his instructions regarding patient treatment and care.[76] When Sister St. Robitaille retired as administrator of the Blood Hospital in 1931, Dr. Stone expressed his regret over her departure, for he considered her responsible for the success of the hospital.[77]

A great deal of the nurses' time was still consumed by patient care at the Blood and Blackfoot hospitals. When reserve hospitals were renovated, separate TB wards with open-air balconies were built to accommodate patients' treatment. The nurses who worked on these wards on a daily basis faced a particular set of challenges. They were responsible for attending patients with TB; furthermore, it was not unusual for them to develop TB themselves in the course of their work. The sisters at the Blood Hospital were often confined and treated for TB. In a report to the reverend general of the Sisters of Charity at Nicolet in 1924, Dr. Kennedy discussed the state of the nuns' health. He advised that Sister St. Margaret be sent back to Nicolet because she had TB and her condition was not improving. In addition, he noted that Sister Cartier had been bedridden for two months because of a tubercular spot on her lung but would be able to carry on with her duties in another four or five months. He feared that Sister Mary, while not yet sick, would soon fall ill because she had been working far too hard and looked miserable, thin, and worn out. Kennedy wanted the reverend general to persuade Sister Mary to take things easier.[78]

Other continuities emerged in hospital maintenance and the social services provided by Euro-Canadian women. Keeping hospitals clean – a duty made far easier after the hospital renovations – remained a great source of pride among Euro-Canadian health workers and DIA personnel. Medical officers often noted the spotless condition of the Blood Hospital.[79] In a report to the DIA in 1926, the Indian agent at the Blackfoot Reserve, George Gooderham, noted with pride that Matron Alexander kept the hospital spotless and insisted on a systemized condition of affairs.[80] He also noted that the hospitals continued to supply outpatients and visitors to the dispensary with necessary meals. In 1924 the sister superior at the Blood Hospital requested a new oven on the grounds that they were providing up to fifty meals a day for outpatients and that a "considerable number of old people were provided with a daily hot meal" during the winter.[81] Even at the Sarcee Reserve, where there was no formal hospital, the nurse hired by the DIA made efforts whenever possible to supply food from the school to patients at the reserve.[82] The female health workers continued to provide reserve residents with food throughout this period.

Greater differences among female health workers emerged after 1915 and centred on the training and skills nurses were expected to possess. The Euro-Canadian women hired on a temporary basis by the DIA to deal with specific medical situations all possessed formal training, and so too did travelling public health nurses. But far fewer travelling public health nurses were employed, and they worked for much shorter periods of time than their church-affiliated counterparts. Before 1920 many of the women who worked in church-run institutions did not have formal nursing credentials. DIA facilities were therefore run by women of varying expertise and knowledge. After 1920, nurses who worked in DIA hospitals, school infirmaries, and dispensaries were expected to be graduate nurses. In particular, training in obstetrics and knowledge of surgical procedures were necessary qualifications for women who worked in these hospitals. When the Blackfoot Hospital reopened in 1924, its staff consisted of two or three graduate nurses and, as of 1928, a full-time doctor. At the Blood Hospital, this change in staff training was not made until 1927, even though nurses' qualifications had been an intermittent source of concern for more than a decade.

Advances in anaesthetic and surgical techniques led to a corresponding demand for nurses who possessed the knowledge required to assist physicians. If or when this became a concern at the Blackfoot Hospital is not revealed in the records. At the Blood Hospital, however, the negotiation that resulted in an understanding of the skills sisters were required to possess is plainly laid out. Questions were first raised about the sisters' lack of formal credentials by Dr. Edwards, medical officer for the Kainai, in late 1912. When he learned that the sisters were unable to admit maternity cases or treat female patients suffering from any "illnesses peculiar to women," he immediately brought the matter to the DIA's attention.[83] Steps to address this concern were not immediately taken. After the First World War, however, the practical nursing skills and experience possessed by the Grey Nuns were increasingly regarded as inadequate. Perhaps the growing use of reserve hospitals made their lack of training more visible. This sentiment was expressed by Dr. Kennedy, the Blood Reserve's medical officer, in a letter to the superior general at Nicolet in 1927:

> We are getting more patients and more serious cases and I will say that with some of the serious cases, the sisters are not able to properly look after them. They do their best, and are willing in every sense, but they lack the necessary knowledge, training and experience; they are not trained as nurses and as a result the patients suffer unnecessarily. Furthermore, any number of times, I would operate at the hospital but cannot do so because I have not the necessary trained assistance ... There is not one single sister who has had any surgical training; none who can give anesthetic, or can be trusted to do so; and none whom I can depend upon to assist at any operation, no matter how small.[84]

Dr. Kennedy wanted the mother house to supply at least three graduate nurses with training in surgery, obstetrics, and general medicine. Nurses were now expected to possess skills that reflected advances in scientific medical knowledge.[85]

This change was echoed in the proliferation of DIA hospitals in the Treaty 7 area and in the movement of reserve health care services from informal or domestic to institutional settings. At the insistence of the Kainai, Dr. Kennedy, and the sister superior, the mother house sent two sisters with formal nurse training to the Blood Hospital.

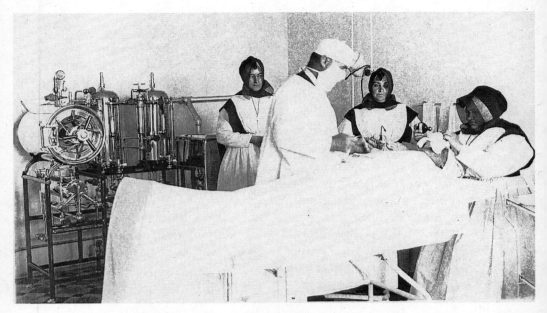

Grey Nuns assisting the DIA medical officer in surgery at the Blood Hospital, Cardston, Alberta, 1930s. | Courtesy Grey Nuns Archives, Montreal

Tensions within DIA Institutions

Nurses' work at reserve hospitals increasingly came under the supervision of doctors, Indian agents, and nursing supervisors, usually called matrons. Miss Alexander was appointed the matron of the Blackfoot Hospital after it was renovated. In 1928 the hospital acquired a full-time physician, Dr. Evelyn Windsor. From this point on, descriptions of nurses' work began to include accounts of the assistance they gave DIA doctors, which indicates a decline in the autonomy of female workers. Doctors resented the intrusion of other authorities when they performed procedures. This was the case when the doctor for the Blood Hospital complained heatedly in a letter to the department that he and the matron had been performing a procedure when a priest came along and pulled her away. The doctor became incensed further when the matron did not return to complete her task.[86] Nurses were subject to multiple and often competing levels of authority within the hospital.

It was at the Blood Reserve, where two churches were competing for souls, that religion became the biggest source of tension. During the late

1920s, the religious affiliation of the staff running the Blood Hospital became a growing source of conflict both within the DIA and between the Anglicans and the Catholics at the reserve. These tensions, however, were not high enough for the DIA to end its relationship with the sisters. The nuns, after all, were willing to work for very little. In 1931 the department paid the Sisters of Charity a grand total of $340 per month for eight sisters – three of whom were graduate nurses. The sisters' vows of poverty and charity made the meagre pay and primitive living quarters tolerable.[87]

Religious friction at the Blood Reserve reached its height in the 1920s during negotiations for a new hospital at Cardston. The issue was who would run the hospital. When the DIA decided to build a new hospital in 1928, the Anglicans vied with the Roman Catholics for the right to staff and operate the facility.[88] The acrimony between the two churches had been festering for years. The Anglicans made surprise visits to the Blood Hospital to inspect it for problems.[89] In response, the sisters encouraged their Roman Catholic supporters at the reserve to forward letters and petitions of support to the federal government. In May 1927 three members of the Kainai band council sent a petition in support of the sisters' work and requested that the nuns be kept on to run the new hospital.[90]

Frustrated by the complaints, the Indian agent at the Blood Reserve suggested that it would be best for the department and the community to establish a non-denominational hospital.[91] The DIA concurred but was unwilling to relinquish the affordable labour provided by the nursing sisters.[92] Department officials therefore wrote up a series of regulations that outlined the future operations of the hospital and the conduct of its staff. These regulations drew clear distinctions between the caring and curative labour of the sisters as nurses and their religious work as nuns. The regulations forbade clergy of any denomination from living in the hospital, and no religious emblems or pictures were to be displayed on the outside of the building or in any room or place used for patients or visitors. If a patient required the immediate services of a clergyman, the Indian agent was to be told so he could notify the appropriate people. In addition, clergy of all denominations would be free to conduct religious services and ministrations in the hospital.[93]

This last regulation applied only to recognized Western religions, not to Aboriginal religious practices. The Grey Nuns regarded these rules as hostile to their congregation and antithetical to their work. In their view the point of the regulations was to limit their role as missionaries.[94] Indeed, the General Council at Nicolet voted unanimously to reject the regulations and withdraw their congregation from the Blood Reserve if a compromise

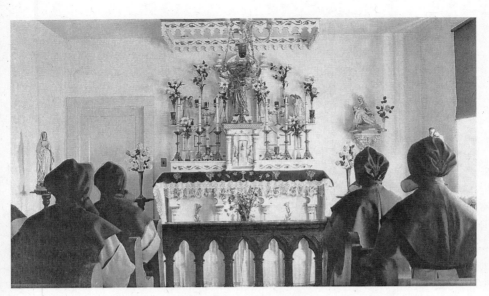

The chapel at the new Blood Hospital, Cardston, Alberta, 1930s. | Courtesy Grey Nuns Archives, Montreal

could not be negotiated. John Kidd, the bishop of Calgary, was able to convince the sisters to remain at their mission. He was certain that over time they would once again be able to operate freely in the institution.[95] This optimism proved to be unfounded.

Another source of conflict between the Grey Nuns and the department involved staff changes at the Blood Hospital. According to the constitution of the Sisters of Charity, a new sister superior was to be elected by the reverend general and the General Council every three years.[96] When Sister St. Robitaille retired in 1931, after serving an unprecedented nine years as sister superior at the Blood Hospital, her departure was not well received by Dr. Harold McGill, head of the IHS.[97] When her replacement, Sister Mary, was in turn replaced in 1934, McGill sent another angry letter to the reverend general: "I wish to point out," he complained, "that it is not the Department's intention that this should invest your Order with the privilege of changing the Superior without due arrangement and authority."[98] Exchanges of this sort reflected growing discord between the Grey Nuns and the department. The Grey Nuns were accustomed to greater autonomy and felt that the DIA was hostile to their congregation and that its criticisms were a sign that IHS was trying to replace Grey Nuns with Protestant staff.[99]

Travelling Nurses and Public Health Instruction

After 1915 the DIA continued to strengthen its grip on the IHS and to centralize its bureaucracy. These developments and the founding of a travelling-nurse program in 1922 mirrored changes in health services in Euro-Canadian communities in southern Alberta. Medical services in those communities expanded throughout the early twentieth century. After Alberta became a province in 1905, it gained control over its own public health services. In 1906 it appointed its first medical officer of health, Dr. A.E. Clendennan. Over the next ten years, the province established a public health bureaucracy of boards, laws, regulations, and laboratories. In 1917 Alberta became the second province to implement a Municipal Hospitalization Plan, which was partly funded by taxes. Under that plan, standard ward care was offered at one dollar a day.[100] In 1919 the province founded a Department of Public Health.

Despite these developments, consistent medical care remained beyond the reach of many Euro-Canadians in rural Alberta. In 1919 the Alberta District Nursing Service was founded to meet the needs for midwifery and emergency medical services in rural communities.[101] In 1920 the first Child Welfare Clinic was established in Edmonton, and similar clinics soon opened in Calgary, Medicine Hat, Drumheller, and Vegerville.[102] By 1922 the Alberta District Nursing Service comprised twelve rural districts staffed by thirty public health nurses. That same year the DIA hired four public health nurses to administer all of the reserves in the three Prairie provinces. The public health nurses hired by the Alberta government were involved in a number of programs that ranged from prenatal and postnatal advice, school health services, and home visits to health and home-nursing lectures.

Hard times in the early 1920s forced the United Farmers of Alberta (UFA) government to cut its funding of health services and to create a 50/50 cost-sharing program with local municipalities.[103] As a result, many of the programs offered by district health nurses were sharply curtailed, and services were dramatically reduced. The number of public health nurses dropped to six by 1925.[104] The non-Aboriginal population of Alberta, according to the 1921 census, was around 575,000.[105] It thus seemed that Treaty 7 nations, which had one travelling nurse for roughly four thousand people, now enjoyed a better nurse-to-patient ratio.[106]

Mobile travelling clinics were introduced in rural Alberta in the summer of 1924 in an effort to address the shortage of health services, especially for children, in many rural communities. These clinics provided a variety of services such as general physical examinations, tonsillectomies, minor operations, vaccinations, and dental care.[107] They operated each summer from 1924 to 1933. The clinics usually spent two days at one site, and people would come from all over the district to be examined and treated. Some settlers remembered travelling thirty to forty miles in horse-drawn wagons to take advantage of these clinics' services.[108] The clinics did not extend their services to communities in which medical or dental help was already available. The need for travelling clinics declined during the 1930s in response to falling infant and maternal mortality rates.[109]

A similar process took place at reserves after 1915. The role of visiting or public health nurses became more significant. Although efforts to inculcate Aboriginal women with appropriate feminine and domestic arts had been made by Euro-Canadian missionary women before 1915, after 1915 these schemes were more explicitly tied to concerns about health and sanitation. For example, mothering classes and baby shows linked household management and child care practices to ill health and high infant mortality rates. The role of female health workers as agents of social change took on new meaning.[110]

The belief that Aboriginal women were negligent mothers and indifferent to the health of their children was reflected in policies developed by the DIA and in the tasks that Euro-Canadian women were hired to perform. For example, in 1914 the DIA created the position of field matron, even though local farmer's wives had been hired as field matrons in western Canada as early as 1905.[111] In the department's annual report for 1923, Duncan Campbell Scott defines the duties of field matrons as follows: "Encourage the Indian women and girls to make their homes more like those of white people. Instead of thinking only of daily needs, they are being taught to provide for the future ... It is felt that by such simple instruction in the art of living coupled with care given by the Indian Agents and medical attendants, the health of the Indian people [will] be material[ly] improved."[112]

Travelling nurses were meant to supplement field matrons' work with public health initiatives. As discussed earlier in this chapter, the duties of travelling nurses included providing therapeutic services wherever and whenever they were required. Equally important, however, was their supervisory and educational labour. They were to give talks on sanitation, nutrition, homemaking, and child care. They were also expected to set up monthly baby clinics and hold baby shows to "stimulate Indian parents in the proper method of caring for their children."[113] It is not known how often these clinics were held, but given the large population these women administered, it is quite likely they were sporadic. Nurses were also expected to encourage Aboriginal women to cultivate gardens and to instruct them in canning and preserving vegetables. The point was to teach Aboriginal women how to plan for the future.[114]

Initiatives such as these reflected the growing influence of social reformers and scientific motherhood in Canadian society. The burgeoning fields of domestic science and home economics shaped how the DIA – and Euro-Canadian society more broadly – viewed women's roles as household managers and mothers. The application of scientific principles to household management implied that there were precise and predictable rules to order domestic space. Women who adhered to these rules were seen as ensuring the health and well-being of their families.[115] Department officials therefore believed that Aboriginal women's capacity to improve their communities lay in their domestic and mothering abilities. Links were being forged in the minds of policy-makers between domestic health and women's so-called natural roles as nurturers and mothers. The DIA's annual report for 1903 identifies domestic virtues as "at the root of all national greatness [and this was shown in a woman's] desire to improve the home surroundings."[116] The department maintained that the character of Aboriginal dwellings was closely related to the overall well-being of the community.[117] According to the officials, ill health was a result of poor cooking methods, lack of proper domestic space, the failure to segregate the sexes, dirt floors, the want of appropriate furniture, and poor housekeeping. It therefore sought to address these problems through legislation, surveillance, coercion, and instructional programs.[118]

Besides their nursing duties, Euro-Canadian women after 1915 were required to inspect residents' homes, keep track of expectant mothers and their children, and provide instruction in home care, cooking, child care, and sanitation. By doing so, female health care workers became part of the state's apparatus for classifying Aboriginal culture. Historian John Lutz contends that the tabulation of annual censuses was not simply about demography and economic statistics: it was also about "moral statistics, which would measure, in an approximate way, the morality and civilization of Aboriginal people."[119] In other words, a symbolic relationship existed between poor health, high infant morality rates, and Aboriginal women's failure to use Western medicine. The DIA offered the death statistics for Aboriginal children as proof of poor mothering and indifferent parenting. Euro-Canadian women were instrumental in locating, describing, and attempting to rectify problems associated with poor environmental conditions, and Aboriginal women were identified as the root of the problem.

The Indian agent at the Blackfoot Reserve, George Gooderham, required nurses to make certain that patients properly followed medical advice. In 1925, when a whooping cough epidemic broke out at that reserve, he sent nurses to remain in the homes of sick people "where it [was] known that the treatment, as set out by the doctor, [was] not be[ing] carried out. While there [the nurse] controls the situation."[120] DIA officials often criticized Aboriginal people for failing to follow the advice of medical officers and, in their view, this resistance justified coercive measures such as the 1914 amendment to the Indian Act. Department officials believed that Aboriginal parents – mothers especially – were utterly incapable of caring properly for their families. In her study of health and architecture, Annmarie Adams contends that the "house and body were inextricably linked, and [when women ensured] the well-being of domestic spaces [they ensured] the health of the inhabitants of that space."[121] As evidence, the department pointed to high infant morbidity rates and the reluctance of Aboriginal homemakers to model themselves on middle-class Euro-Canadians. According to DIA officials, the failure of Aboriginal women to adopt Western cultural norms was reflected in their slovenly homes, poorly prepared meals, and shoddily dressed children.[122] To change the situation, Scott recommended that Aboriginal mothers be rewarded for successfully rearing their children to a certain age.

The nurse stationed permanently at the Stoney Reserve in 1927-28 echoed DIA officials when she blamed Aboriginal parents when their children died.[123] The Indian agent, Robert Pringle, shared the nurse's view and noted that eleven children had died and that the parents could be blamed for not requesting a doctor. That is, he blamed the superstition and ignorance of Nakoda mothers who rejected Western biomedicine and relied on "old squaws": "The Indians have been told hundreds of times that when anyone is sick to come to the office and ask for the doctor, but there was not a single parent ... who notified the office ... I have questioned the parents and they claim that the children all had sufficient clothing when they were taken out, but that may have not been so ... The parents should be punished in some way for not reporting the sickness but it is pretty hard to prove neglect."[124] Pringle went so far as to suggest that Aboriginal parents be penalized (even further) for the deaths of their children.[125]

Part of the nurse's mandate at Morley was to keep a register of expectant mothers so that she could "track prospective births [and] make a point of paying frequent visits to the home as the time draws near."[126] The policy reflected a growing effort at the Stoney and Sarcee reserves not only to track the number of children born but also to intervene in childbirth and beyond. Pringle also tried to enlist the aid of the band chief and councillors to report any illnesses to him.[127] The problem, according to the DIA, lay not in the material and social realities of reserves but rather in the neglect and ignorance of Aboriginal parents. Government officials did not try to understand why Nakoda parents hid their children or why they refused the Western medical aid offered by travelling nurses and medical officers. Without a hospital at the Stoney Reserve, perhaps parents were afraid their children would be removed to an off-reserve facility, never to be seen again.

The 1920s witnessed a surge in advice literature directed at women about pregnancy and infant care.[128] The object of this literature was to reinforce "the traditional sexual division of labour in the home, undermine women's autonomy as mothers, and promote standards more in keeping with the values, lifestyles, and resources of its middle class, professional authors, and sponsors than those of its intended audience."[129] This literature normalized unrealistic and culturally irrelevant expectations of non-white mothers and subjected them to even greater scrutiny. In his 1897 annual report to the DIA, Agent Samuel Lucas of the Sarcee Reserve wrote that he believed "the Indians [did] not exercise the least control over their children, they are allowed to go in or out, sick or well, during the most inclement weather, often insufficiently clad."[130] Thomas Graham, the Indian agent at the Peigen Reserve, attributed the death of a child to an inherited lack of stamina and to overfeeding.[131] Department officials maintained that Aboriginal parents were indifferent to the well-being of their children. In their view, this apathy was apparent in Aboriginal parents' failure to properly dress and feed their children and in their refusal to seek out Western physicians to treat sick children.[132]

In 1925, when Duncan Campbell Scott learned that the death rate among the Siksika had been the same as the birth rate, he raised concerns.[133] Gooderham responded by placing the blame squarely on those families of "low vitality where the children did not get the proper care in their homes ... Despite instructions and warnings by the medical officer and others, some Indians, particularly those who are past middle age or are of low mentality, fail to care properly for their children."[134] Scott concurred with Gooderham's assessment and suggested that a system of rewards be instituted to appeal to the maternal instincts of Aboriginal women and "overcome the apathy of the Indians in this matter."[135]

Given the available sources, it is difficult to assess how nurses operated within the DIA's racist discourse. It is clear, though, that some nurses completely endorsed the DIA's perspective. For example, the travelling nurse for southern Alberta complained that the Nakoda could "not be persuaded to give proper care to their children, frequently failing to report the illness of a child until after its death. Some of the Indians even hide their children when they are ill, to avoid treatment by the doctor or nurse."[136] Nurses failed to recognize that when Aboriginal parents hid their children it was because they mistrusted the DIA and its agents, especially when it came to the care of their children. High death rates at the Morley Residential School did not endear the DIA to parents.

But there is also some evidence that nurses tried to make their work more relevant to Treaty 7 nations. There are almost five years of extant monthly reports from the public health nurses hired to work at the Sarcee Reserve from 1915 to 1918. Some nurses were more vigilant than others about visiting the reserve and monitoring the health of mothers and children. For example, Maud Hill, who worked at the Sarcee Reserve in 1917, made frequent visits to Aboriginal homes, was present at the ration house, and was often called by reserve residents during medical emergencies. In contrast, Helen Wright worked for the department briefly and did not push the strict boundaries of her job. Wright remained at the residential school and did not make any trips to the reserve unless specifically called for, which was a rare occurrence. The effectiveness of the DIA's programs depended on the initiative of the individuals who ran them.

Some nurses, such as Hill, energetically performed their work, and their reports offer a wealth of information. Hill's reports show that she focused her efforts on transforming Aboriginal homes and improving the health and care of children. To accomplish this, she acquired a list of those homes with small children and performed monthly inspections.[137] During her visits she provided Aboriginal women with direction as to the "feeding, cleanliness, and care of their children, also advised them as to the washing and airing of bedding and housecleaning."[138] Five months later she submitted another report in which she described her work: "Special visits to eight families consisting of nine boys and four girls. Instructions given as to the care, cleanliness and feeding of young children. Also as to washing and airing of personal clothing and bedding. I have advised the women to protect their food from flies and dust."[139] Hill also made regular maternity visits to pregnant women at the reserve.[140] In fact she was very conscientious about ensuring that women's maternity visits were up to date. She also acknowledged the difficulties that Aboriginal women faced in conforming to Western middle-class ideas about housekeeping when she noted that the frequent scrubbing of women's houses was inhibited by the distance they had to travel to haul water from the creek.[141] The planning of reserve communities had not taken into account the proximity of water. At the Blackfoot Reserve, residents were fortunate enough by 1914 to have one water pump for every three or four groups of houses.[142] By 1916 the Kainai were still obtaining water from the mountain-fed stream that passed by the reserve. It is worth noting that this inconvenient water source probably accounted for the absence of typhoid in the community.[143]

At the Blackfoot Reserve, Miss Alexander, the hospital matron, established baby clinics. Alexander was responsible for "teach[ing] mothers the proper feeding, care and clothing of babies as well as provid[ing] practical demonstrations and advice to mothers to be."[144] As an incentive for Aboriginal mothers to attend the clinics, baby shows were held, with monetary prizes of ten dollars paid out of band funds.[145] Those who judged these shows considered the following: the baby's appearance of health; the presence or absence of physical defects and skin blemishes; cleanliness and neatness of attire; height, weight, chest, and head measurements; and the parents' general approach to caring for the child.[146] Public health nurses and field matrons used these contests to draw tangible links between the instruction they had provided and observable markers of what the DIA identified as progress. Historian Gerald Thomson has identified the Better Baby contests in Vancouver and New Westminster, BC, as "a theatrical means of alerting Anglo-Saxon British Columbians" to racial degeneration.[147] In much the same way, female health workers used baby shows to make Aboriginal people aware of their children's supposed deficiencies.

Miss Annie Brandon, a travelling nurse, had launched a similar program at the Stoney Reserve the previous year with identical objectives. At her first meeting, she gave a talk about "sanitation and prevention of disease by infection and contagion."[148] She declared the program a success because over the course of three months she had encouraged more expectant mothers to be examined by the doctor, had assisted in eleven births, and had been able to show Aboriginal mothers the importance of bathing newborns.[149] She viewed the program's success as a function of the superiority of Western medicine, not as a result of her dedication or character. It is difficult to know how Nakoda women felt about the services and programs offered by female health workers. At times, lay nurses and female medical missionaries unwittingly recorded their responses when they commented on the reactions of Aboriginal women to their presence.

Nurses were not blind to the conditions in which their patients lived. Indeed, there is evidence that female health workers tried to serve as advocates for the people among whom they worked. For instance, in 1924 Miss Brandon, a travelling nurse, reported to the department that she was

Chapter Six

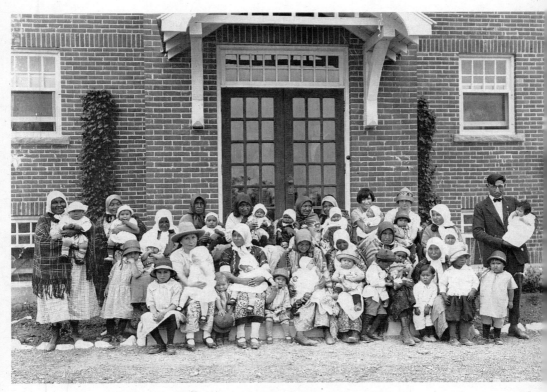

Contestants of the first Baby Show held at the Blackfoot Reserve. The contest was organized by Miss Alexander, the hospital matron, 1926. *Front row, L-R:* Mrs. Charles Joe Royal (1st prize winner), Mrs. Harry Red Gun (2nd prize), and Mrs. A. Youngman (3rd prize). Mrs. Jack McHugh is in the back row, right, in the cloche hat. The man on the extreme right is Earl Calf Child, the Indian agent's interpreter. He is holding the baby of Mrs. Spring Calf, who died in childbirth. The child was raised at the hospital. | Courtesy Glenbow Archives PA-32-1

constantly besieged by complaints from the Kainai that they were not getting enough to eat. She added her own assessment, which concurred with the opinions of the Kainai, and she felt it her duty to mention this matter in her report.[150] When Miss Brandon became aware that the department had taken this matter up with Indian agent Joseph Thomas Faunt, she immediately wrote and apologized for her criticism. She began her letter with a line from a song: "Everybody slips a little now and then?"[151] Brandon's assessment of the situation at the Blood Reserve was accurate, yet she also recognized that her ability to perform her work depended on the co-operation of DIA officials. These checks on the workplace autonomy of female health workers limited their ability to serve as effective advocates for Aboriginal people.

Conclusion

Between 1915 and 1930, the improvised health system started by the churches was gradually taken over by the DIA. Although missionary women continued to be present on reserves, their active roles in healing and nursing care declined. The most obvious exception to this rule was the nuns at the Blood Hospital, who remained until 1954. Many of the lay Euro-Canadian women who took over the curing and caring roles of missionary women spent less time among Aboriginal people and did not remain on any reserve for an extended time. The fiscal conservatism that informed the DIA's programs limited the effectiveness of the field matrons and travelling nurses both as health care practitioners and as agents of social change.

The supposedly poor domestic and mothering skills of Aboriginal women were deemed impediments to the progress of Aboriginal communities. Aboriginal women were blamed for ill health in Aboriginal communities because they lacked the necessary domestic arts and motherly skills. It was therefore seen as the duty of the department – especially its female employees – to teach Aboriginal women about European notions of domesticity and hygiene so they could contribute to the progress of their communities. In the eyes of officials, if Aboriginal women displayed an aptitude for domestic virtues, it would show the department they were willing to participate in the state's efforts to civilize them. Baking bread, making butter, canning fruits and vegetables, and cultivating gardens were seen as recognizable and concrete symbols of Aboriginal women's progress.[152]

The degree to which Euro-Canadian women followed DIA policy directives is difficult to gauge, as is the degree of success they experienced when implementing those directives. Letters of the sort that female missionaries wrote to mission societies describing their activities do not exist for female employees of the DIA. There were times when the concerns of female health care workers for the well-being of their patients came into conflict with departmental policies and directives. The ability of Euro-Canadian women to foster change was limited, and their efforts to do so had the potential to generate tension when proper bureaucratic channels were not followed or when criticisms were levelled at the department. The ability of female personnel to improve conditions on Treaty 7 reserves was severely handicapped by bureaucratic inertia, ambivalence, and unequal gender relations.

Programs run by female missionaries, field matrons, and public health nurses were geared toward encouraging Aboriginal women to adopt middle-class European ideas of housekeeping and child rearing.[153] According to these women, an Aboriginal woman's decision to use Western medicine, especially during pregnancy and childbirth, was tightly linked to her efforts to create an appropriate healthy home environment for her family. Criminologist and historian Mariana Valverde, in her work on moral reform in English Canada, identifies medicine as the practical and symbolic link between personal regeneration and scientific urban reform – or in this case, the reserve environment.[154] Aboriginal women who chose to use Western medicine were symbolically reforming not only themselves but also their physical environment. Hospitals on reserves and their increasing use by reserve residents suggested to department officials the ultimate defeat of traditional Aboriginal culture as epitomized by the existence of the medicine man.[155] Seeking out what was considered appropriate and adequate medical care was central to the idea of responsible motherhood. Western medicine thus became a potent narrative of development, and its use became a standard by which progress was measured. For women, this narrative was constructed according to prevailing concepts of women's roles relating to scientific motherhood, public health, and child care.

Maternity work was emphasized because the roles women performed as mothers were regarded as vital to the progress of Aboriginal peoples and the nation more generally. After the First World War, according to the DIA, all aspects of child care and motherhood in Aboriginal communities were in desperate need of reform. Yet Aboriginal communities continued to resist, as is evident in the perseverance of Aboriginal women's midwifery skills. Although the 1920s witnessed a decline in the number of children born outside DIA hospitals, Aboriginal women continued to draw from the experience and knowledge of midwives and medicine women. Healing and caregiving remained a site of resistance and cultural persistence in Treaty 7 communities.

7
The Snake and the Butterfly
Midwifery and Birth Control, 1900s-30s

Institutional health care, although still somewhat piecemeal, was firmly in place on Treaty 7 reserves by the 1920s. Department of Indian Affairs (DIA) hospitals, public health programs, residential schools, and white female health care personnel were shaping the medical choices made by Aboriginal people, especially women. The number of people who relied on Aboriginal healers declined. But this process was not uniform, and Aboriginal women continued to provide their communities with necessary midwifery services, including contraception. Biomedicine did not replace Aboriginal medicine; instead, medical pluralism was practised. The treatments that were chosen depended on a variety of factors: in some situations, Western medicine was more effective, while in others, Aboriginal medicine was superior. In spite of – or perhaps because of – the state's best efforts, Aboriginal women continued to operate as midwives, healers, and caregivers in southern Alberta.

During the interwar years, the DIA tried harder to control where childbirth took place in Aboriginal communities. Before the First World War, very few Aboriginal women gave birth in reserve hospitals. Most women had their children at home, attended by an experienced midwife, who provided pre- and postnatal care with the support of female family members. The relative success of Aboriginal midwives and structural problems within the DIA health system made childbirth and Aboriginal midwifery a low priority for the department throughout much of this period. The DIA showed little interest in intervening in the birth experiences of Aboriginal women. But by the 1920s, the DIA's policy toward pre- and postnatal care had changed, and the department began trying to induce Aboriginal women to make the transition from deliveries managed by midwives to "physician controlled and hospital-based birth."[1] This trend reflected government policies throughout the West, where women's organizations (such as the United Farm Women of Alberta) were lobbying their provincial governments to address excessively high rates of maternal and infant mortality through broader public health programs. For their part, department officials believed that high infant mortality rates among Aboriginal peoples were not the result of poor access to Western medical care; rather, they were a consequence of Aboriginal women's decisions not to use the Western medical services the department was making available. In the view of officials, the solution to high infant and maternal mortality was to ensure that Aboriginal women were closely monitored by nurses throughout pregnancy, that they gave birth in DIA hospitals or were attended by a graduate nurse, that they were instructed in Euro-Canadian child care methods, and that they were given periodic checkups. Yet, despite the DIA's efforts, Aboriginal women continued to work as midwives and healers for their communities.

In contrast, contraception practices in Treaty 7 communities were entirely overlooked by the DIA throughout this period. The reason for this oversight is not known. By the nineteenth century, non-Aboriginal people were using various forms of contraception to limit family size, as evidenced by declining birth rates among middle-class Euro-Canadians. In addition, industrialization, modernity, and the growing presence of non-British immigrants had moved issues of birth control and abortion to centre stage in Canadian politics. Fears of race suicide even led social reformers to lobby for the criminalization of abortion and birth control under subsection 179c of the 1892 Criminal Code, which would make the dissemination of information about or the procurement of abortion or birth control indictable offences. In other words, discussions about birth control and abortion were prevalent in the late nineteenth and early twentieth centuries, and both topics were viewed as public and moral issues. Why did this not touch Aboriginal people, who had been targets of social and moral correction in every other possible sphere? Perhaps because, for most of that era, they were regarded as a vanishing race – a perception that was only strengthened by the DIA's own reports, which provided statistics that enumerated the ill health of Aboriginal people. Or perhaps at the time the real concern was who was reproducing – in other words, contraception among Aboriginal peoples would only have become a source concern if middle-class European-Canadian women had begun to follow their lead.

Several historians contend that this oversight went much deeper – that it had its roots in the racialized and primitive stereotypes assigned to non-white women in the eighteenth and nineteenth centuries. According to Patricia Jasen, nineteenth-century texts disparaged Aboriginal women by representing them as primitive and animal-like, and these misrepresentations led to a distortion of non-Aboriginal understandings of birth culture in Aboriginal communities. Building on Jasen's work, Maureen Lux contends that the myth that Aboriginal women gave birth painlessly – accepted by most Europeans during the nineteenth century – made the study of midwifery among Aboriginal people seem unnecessary.[2] More recent studies of health in Aboriginal communities focus almost exclusively on death, disease, and the failure of health care regimes to resolve ill health. While all of this is important to acknowledge, the fascination with this culture of death has ensured that midwifery and contraception have been almost entirely overlooked in Aboriginal communities. The weight given to rates of morbidity and mortality, to poor living conditions, and to efforts by DIA employees and missionary organizations to undermine Aboriginal culture have masked the survival of the midwifery and birth control practices of northwestern Plains peoples.

Over the past decade, feminist scholars and community activists have fought to address this oversight, especially within communities that are struggling to reclaim control over the birth process. Works by Betty-Anne Daviss and John O'Neil and Patricia Kaufert, for example, confront the misconceptions surrounding Aboriginal childbirth practices by acknowledging the extensive tradition of midwifery in Inuit communities.[3] Historical studies of midwifery acknowledge the regional, ethnic, and racial variations that have existed in both the practice and the decline of midwifery throughout Canada. In less settled regions of Canada, for example, midwifery persisted far longer than in urban and industrialized centres such as Toronto.[4] The growth of this literature, and of interest in the topic, paralleled the re-emergence of a movement in the late 1980s and 1990s to legalize midwifery in Canada.[5] Aboriginal birthing culture (centred on the medicine woman and experienced older women) has become a model from which midwifery activists can now draw in their efforts to de-medicalize childbirth and make it a more female-centred experience. Yet, in spite of public acceptance and the passage of midwifery legislation in recent years, the "dominant Canadian model of midwifery endorsed [remains] to a large extent ill-suited for counterparts in Aboriginal communities" because this paradigm remains rooted in Western models of midwifery from countries such as Britain.[6] This chapter builds on this literature by showing that the midwifery work of Aboriginal women was not something that re-emerged; rather, it persisted throughout the period under examination and is emblematic of the resilience of Aboriginal culture and the importance of women's knowledge and work in their communities.

Hospital Births

Throughout the period of this study, DIA reports and correspondence characterized Aboriginal medicine as a pervasive problem in Treaty 7 communities. But a focus on the more public – and typically masculine – elements of Aboriginal medicine meant that less visible and feminine curative practices, including midwifery, were often overlooked. It was not until the 1920s – when studies revealed high infant and maternal mortality rates among Canadian women, especially in the West – that Aboriginal midwifery was regarded as a problem and that concerted efforts were made to encourage doctor- or nurse-assisted births in Aboriginal communities. In her examination of northwestern Plains women and the formulation of DIA policy, historian Pamela White argues that the First World War was a watershed in the federal government's struggle to refashion Aboriginal motherhood.[7] This transformation, combined with more general concerns relating to the health of the Canadian population, intersected with the DIA's agenda to promote Euro-Canadian–style domesticity on reserves.[8]

The welfare of children and infants came to be synonymous with the health and well-being of mothers.[9] According to nursing historian Sharon Richardson, a study performed by the federal government during the early 1920s revealed that Alberta had the highest maternal mortality rates in the country and that maternity was the second-leading cause of death among women in the nation.[10] In 1919, as a direct result of persistent lobbying by women's groups, the Alberta District Nursing Service was established to provide midwifery and emergency medical services to isolated communities.[11] These efforts reflected a growing belief among the Euro-Canadian medical community that women required professional medical personnel to deliver babies, if not from doctors then from nurses with obstetrical training.

In reserve communities, efforts to monitor expectant mothers, alter the location of births, and intervene in delivery were not significant until the 1920s. The DIA's ambivalence about intervening in the obstetrical world of Aboriginal women was a result of three factors. First, racist stereotypes that characterized the childbirth experience of Aboriginal women as painless owing to their uncivilized nature made biomedical intervention by the state seem pointless.[12] Second, and more significantly, the relative success of Aboriginal midwives during the period of this study made the involvement of nurses and physicians unnecessary for Aboriginal women. For Aboriginal women, hospital birth started to become appealing only after nurses began to permit children to stay at the hospital with their mothers and after advances in asepsis and surgical techniques dramatically improved women's chances of survival. Third and finally, some DIA institutions such as the Blood Hospital simply lacked the resources to deal with maternity cases until 1918.

It was not until the interwar period that non-Aboriginal women began entering hospitals to give birth. Before the First World War, hospitals were generally regarded as places where poor people went to die or be quarantined. Individuals who could afford medical and nursing care remained at home. The transition from home care to hospital care in Canada took place gradually between 1890 and 1920. As historians David Gagan and Rosemary Gagan argue, the "rise of the modern public hospital as a doctor's workshop of medical science for all members of the community [took place] between 1920 and 1950."[13] Few women, if they could help it, gave birth in hospitals until after the Second World War. In Alberta – a province that was predominantly rural until after 1945 – the role of midwives, home remedies, and experienced and helpful female neighbours persisted much longer than in more urban and industrial areas of the country.

During the 1920s the DIA drew a clear link between high infant and maternal mortality rates and the failure of Aboriginal women to use hospital facilities. When an Aboriginal woman died from postpartum complications after giving birth at her home in 1926, Dr. Alan Kennedy blamed the woman and her family for choosing not to attend the hospital.[14] Although Kennedy had been called to help this woman, he had refused to do so while the woman remained at home. The woman died. In a letter of explanation written to Indian agent Joseph Thomas Faunt, Kennedy expressed his hope that this incident would serve both as a lesson and as a reminder to the Kainai about the dangers of having babies at home. Since most Euro-Canadian women continued to give birth at home during this period, it is clear that Kennedy referred in particular to the homes of Aboriginal people. According to historian Wendy Mitchinson, most women who had babies in hospitals during this period were poor or single.[15] Moreover, Aboriginal women were identified as a high-risk group despite the presence of significant familial support. Working-class women faced similar criticisms from middle-class reformers and public health campaigns.[16] The DIA most likely knew that many Aboriginal women chose to be attended by Aboriginal midwives and believed that altering the location of the birth, from the home to the hospital, would help end this practice.

Aboriginal women in the Treaty 7 area did not choose to go to department hospitals in great numbers until the 1920s. During interviews she conducted with Aboriginal women, historian Maureen Lux learned that some women started to use hospitals because few experienced midwives were available on reserves by the late 1920s. Attendance at residential schools had prevented young women from participating in the apprenticeship process and interrupted the intergenerational transfer of knowledge. Other women simply wanted to have "their babies in the new way."[17] Public health campaigns carried out on reserves and in residential schools by nurses and field matrons clearly influenced the choices made by some Aboriginal women, especially those coming out of the residential schools.

The true impact of the state's efforts to control childbirth for Aboriginal women during this period is difficult to gauge. The number of Aboriginal midwives who possessed the necessary obstetrical expertise might well have diminished in southern Alberta after 1900. Oral interviews conducted in the early 1990s with Treaty 7 elders who were born between 1905 and 1934 indicated that, although people continued to be born at home during this period, the work of graduate and public health nurses, field matrons, and nursing sisters had an effect. Of the 200 elders interviewed, 142 offered some details regarding the circumstances of their birth. Between 1905 and 1934, 85 of them were born at home, while 57 were born in hospital. Before 1920, only 6 people interviewed were born in hospital. After 1920, 43 were born at home compared to 45 who were born in hospital under the supervision of doctor or a nurse with obstetrical training.[18] Clearly, the number of people born in a Western medical facility began to increase after 1920.

Other factors influenced Aboriginal women's childbirth choices. George Gooderham, Indian agent at the Blackfoot Reserve, believed that their reluctance to be attended by a white male doctor was a major reason why they did not use the hospital for maternity care. The normative standards that were being developed for labour and childbirth – for example, regarding the appropriate length of labour and its various stages – required that women's childbirth experiences conform to certain expectations. Historian Wendy Mitchinson's thorough study of the history of childbirth outlines some of the changes doctors instituted. For example, they introduced changes to birthing positions that were convenient for doctors but not beneficial for women.[19] Aboriginal women viewed childbirth as a natural process, and imposing normative standards on it would have seemed ridiculous to them. Many of them were accustomed to a female-centred experience, during which a skilled midwife was assisted by the woman's female family members, and would have been uncomfortable with the help of an unfamiliar white male doctor. Indeed, Gooderham contended that it was the arrival of Dr. Evelyn Windsor in 1928, as the full-time medical officer for the hospital, that prompted more Aboriginal women to use the hospital for childbirth.[20]

When Aboriginal women chose to use DIA facilities, it was for their own reasons. Miss Pesquot, a Siksika woman who worked at the Blackfoot Hospital, told anthropologists Jane Richardson and Lucien Hanks that "women seldom come in during the summer for childbirth" and only used the hospital during the winter because it was warmer.[21] The seasonal nature of institutional births is substantiated by the Blood Hospital's records. In 1923 there were three confinements during October, two in December, three in January, and five in March, but only one each in July and August.[22] It seems that hospital facilities were more appealing during the cold winter months.

Until the 1920s, Indian agents would comment – often with surprise – on how rarely white doctors assisted Aboriginal women during childbirth. This can be attributed in part to the continued success of Aboriginal midwives and in part to structural problems in certain DIA institutions. For example, the Roman Catholic Church did not allow the Grey Nuns to treat maternity cases or any "illnesses peculiar to women." For that reason, until December 1918 there were no staff for obstetrical work at the Blood Hospital, nor was that facility equipped for such work.[23] The pope had issued a decree in 1860 that prohibited nuns from performing any work that brought them into the "immediate care of children in the cradle or of women who have children in the houses called maternities."[24] When the Sisters of Charity had volunteered to run the Blood Hospital in the 1890s, this proscription had not troubled department officials. Several decades later, however, when Aboriginal midwives continued to monopolize this particular field of health care and worries about high infant mortality rates were becoming a source of public concern, the department turned its attention to the sisters and the place of childbirth at the Blood Hospital.

Aboriginal midwives continued to practise at Treaty 7 reserves. According to Indian agent W. Julius Hyde, in 1913 Aboriginal midwives were "extremely successful and have prov[en] quite a thorn in Dr. O.C. Edward's side."[25] In 1913 the Blood Hospital was not well attended and with regard to childbirth was not attended at all. If a local midwife was unavailable, reserve residents often elected to travel to Lethbridge or Fort Macleod instead of using the DIA hospital. The department viewed this as the result of two factors: the continued work of Aboriginal medical practitioners, who were preventing women from seeking out proper medical care, and the nuns' lack of formal nursing training.[26] Because the department wanted the Blood Hospital to become a place where expectant mothers could receive proper prenatal and obstetrical care, it entered into protracted negotiations with the sisters and eventually agreed to build a separate maternity ward and pay the salary of a lay graduate nurse to care for confinement cases.[27]

The maternity ward was built in 1916, although it did not open until December 1918.[28] The Roman Catholic Church was extremely reluctant to hire a lay nurse. The sisters felt that a lay woman in their community would be a serious intrusion.[29] Bishop Émile Legal of St. Albert believed that the work of a lay graduate nurse would reflect poorly on the skills of the nursing sisters and that in some situations a lay nurse might challenge the manner in which the nuns carried out their work. He cautioned the reverend general to tread carefully in this matter because he did not want the church to appear to be against progress, especially when it came to its work among Aboriginal peoples. According to the bishop, Catholic hospitals had to change with the times, and many Catholic hospitals already required their sisters to obtain formal training.[30] Because he was determined to ensure that the staff at the Blood Hospital would not appear less competent than their lay counterparts, he suggested that several of the sisters be sent to Calgary for training.[31] A sister from Holy Cross Hospital in Calgary who had experience in maternity cases and who was willing to transgress papal law was eventually sent to the Blood Hospital.[32]

The papal law that prohibited nuns from touching the bodies of women who were pregnant or in labour was finally revoked in 1936, in response to petitions from female Catholic medical missionaries who were genuinely concerned about the health of Aboriginal women and who wanted to make obstetrical care available to the women among whom they worked.[33] In her study of the Catholic Maternity Institute in Santa Fe, New Mexico, Laura Ettinger notes that after 1936 the Roman Catholic Church saw maternity work as a means to reach and save vulnerable mothers and their children, who were potential converts, and to combat the work of Protestant mission groups, which had been offering obstetrical services for decades.[34]

Examining the place of, or lack of, obstetrics in DIA medical facilities is one way to measure the persistence of Aboriginal midwifery. A second method is to examine the use of Aboriginal midwives by missionaries and settlers (see Chapter 3) in an era when Aboriginal cultural practices were supposedly being eradicated. A third approach is to examine personal narratives that were collected by anthropologists in the 1930s alongside the reminiscences of Aboriginal women that have been passed down through oral history or recorded and published.

Descriptions of the work of Aboriginal midwives can be found in the field notes of anthropologists Lucien and Jane Richardson Hanks and Esther Goldfrank, who worked among the Siksika during the summers of 1938 and 1939. A number of people that the Hanks and Goldfrank spoke to emphasized the ongoing importance of Aboriginal midwives in their communities. Indeed, several important aspects of childbirth culture among Plains peoples become clear from the interviews these anthropologists conducted: the existence of a tradition of obstetrical knowledge practised by a medicine woman or midwife, the attendance during the birth of female family members who were familiar with childbirth, and the supportive presence of an experienced woman after the birth to help the new mother become comfortable with her responsibilities. Mary White's story reveals several of these features: "[during the labour] the mother, mother in law and any near female relatives of the expectant mother are supposed to be present. A medicine woman may be called in to ease the labour. One woman holds the arms, another kneads the abdomen gently and the third delivers the child. The mother used to be kept awake for four days, turned constantly to prevent the 'blood from clotting.'"[35]

Jessie, one of Goldfrank's informants, recalled the central role played by Mrs. Scraping White, a medicine woman, during her first pregnancy.[36] Mrs. Scraping White was the first person to examine Jessie and inform her she was pregnant. She then attended Jessie during the birth and remained with Jessie until she was comfortable nursing her son, Sam. Recent oral history accounts suggest that midwives were very important in educating new mothers and often developed lasting relationships with the family.[37]

In the early 1920s, anthropologist Diamond Jenness observed that experienced women among the Tsuu T'ina were well respected for their knowledge and work: "[The] first pangs of labour drove the mother into a separate tent, and brought to her aid three or four old women, one of them a medicine-woman."[38] Obviously, Aboriginal communities had established mechanisms for helping women during and after childbirth. Medicine women gave expectant mothers "a decoction of boiled herbs" to ease the delivery.[39] During the birth of Jessie's first child, her midwife,

Mrs. Scraping Wolf, rubbed a painkiller on her belly to ease her labour. Unfortunately, it was not recorded which plants were used to reduce pain during labour.[40]

Beverly Hungry Wolf interviewed her grandmother, AnadaAki, during the late 1970s. AnadaAki's first childbirth experience reflected many of the same approaches that were recorded in the 1930s: familial support, the presence of a medicine woman, medicinal plant use, and midwifery skills:

> I went into labour at night. I kept on with it all the next day, that night, and on through the morning. It must have been near noon when the baby was born we had our Indian doctors around, and they made brews for us ... I started to feel good and cheerful. Right after the baby was born and taken care of, my mother started to clean me. After I was cleaned she started massaging my bones back into place. I was given some broth to drink and then she laid me down to rest ... During this period of confinement the new mother was bathed and given a cleansing ceremony every four days. Her mother would wash her and then cover her up with a blanket ... To bring the mother's body back to shape in addition to massages, she was made to wear a "belt" or girdle of rawhide.[41]

Aboriginal women had a strong support network and an extensive foundation of knowledge to deal with the childbirth experience. Additional examples come from interviews conducted with Treaty 7 elders in the 1990s. Agnes Red Crow recalled that she had been born at home in a tent surrounded by her grandmothers, who were present to assist her mother.[42] Frank Eagle Tail Feathers remembered that he had been born at home on March 3, 1918, and that his mother had been attended by "some elderly women who were midwives."[43] Allan Shade's mother had a similar experience. His mother had been cared for by his great-grandmothers, who were also midwives.[44] These interviews with Treaty 7 elders reveal that, until 1920, childbirth continued to take place in the home in the presence of female family members.[45] Out of the 94 Treaty 7 elders interviewed who were born between 1920 and 1934, 43 had been born at home, attended by midwives.[46]

In other instances, women chose not to submit entirely to Western medical authority when other options were available. When one of Esther Goldfrank's informants, Violet, gave birth to her first child, Mary, she was treated by the DIA doctor at the Blackfoot Hospital.[47] She had no difficulties during the birth but, one month later, she had problems with her breast and was forced to have it lanced by the doctor. She spent two months in the hospital recovering.[48] Finally, she became impatient and decided to leave. Although the wound had not yet healed, she felt much happier at home and began to recover. Mrs. Sorrel Horse, a medicine woman, treated Violet, and her mother, Jessie, nursed the baby until Violet's breast was healed properly.[49] This type of aftercare, provided by Mrs. Sorrel Horse and Jessie, was essential for the recovery of both mother and child. It is easy to understand why the department had limited success in altering the choices women made about birth attendants.

Birth Control

One facet of Aboriginal women's obstetrical knowledge that was not threatened by DIA medical and educational institutions during this period was their ability to control fertility. Information about contraception was not offered to Aboriginal women by Euro-Canadian women or DIA officers. Neither was access to contraceptives. As mentioned earlier, falling birth rates during the nineteenth century were a clear indication that methods to limit conception were available and in use, but very few Euro-Canadian women were willing to talk publicly about such practices.[50] Even fewer doctors were willing to provide female patients with birth control information, for doing so was an indictable offence under the Criminal Code. Wealthier people could purchase contraceptives from "under the counter of a friendly pharmacist, or they could obtain materials for homemade birth control methods through department store mail order catalogues."[51] It is therefore likely that the health care practitioners who came to work on Treaty 7 reserves and in DIA institutions either knew very little about birth control or feared the legal consequences of disseminating such information.

Yet the unpublished field notes of the ethnographers who studied northwestern Plains peoples during the early twentieth century contain a wealth of information about contraceptive practices. Clark Wissler, for instance, did not discuss these practices in his published works, but his correspondence with David C. Duvall includes many references to birth control. In a letter to Wissler, Duvall writes that quite a few women and some men still had the power to prevent women from having children.[52] According to Duvall, Siksika medicine women, to prevent conception, gave their patients a bracelet or piece of clothing to wear next to their skin, had them stand over a smudge of sweetgrass at night just before they went to bed, and had their bodies painted all over with red ochre.[53] Women were also given something to wear around their neck or waist as a belt, and these objects had a symbol of a snake or butterfly inscribed on them. The Siksika regarded the snake and the butterfly as powerful agents for preventing conception and for expelling the fetus from the womb when it had died during labour.[54]

Esther Goldfrank, in the late 1930s, was one of the first female anthropologists to study the Siksika. Her informant Violet told her that a woman who no longer wanted to have children would visit a medicine woman, who would "tie her up."[55] Children, according to Violet, came from the power of the snake. A medicine woman could therefore prevent conception by tying a snake skin around the woman's waist.[56] Medicine women would often also counsel menstruating women to paint their stomachs with yellow paint.[57]

Claude Schaeffer, another anthropologist who worked in southern Alberta during the 1930s, recorded a wealth of material about Aboriginal birth control practices, although he never published his work. For example, he interviewed Mrs. Victor Chief Coward and recorded that she, after having three children, had sought out Mrs. Mountain Sheep Woman to prevent any further pregnancies. Mrs. Mountain Sheep, whose power to prevent conception came from the rattlesnake and the otter, instructed Mrs. Chief Coward to bathe in a creek, stand over a smudge, and paint her face with yellow earth paint during the first new moon each month (i.e., the time of ovulation).[58] Mrs. Chief Coward followed these instructions for eighteen months before she stopped, "knowing [there was] no chance for further pregnancies."[59] The medicine woman had also given her a bracelet made of otter skin with a figure of a snake drawn on the inside to wear during the new moon. Schaeffer also interviewed Jappy Takes Gun On Top, the only man he encountered who practised birth control medicine. Takes Gun On Top's power to prevent conception was derived from the snake in the form of a beaded necklace.[60]

The prescriptions outlined by Violet, Mrs. Mountain Sheep Woman, and Takes Gun On Top were similar: every month during the full moon, women were to bathe in a creek, stand over a smudge of sweetgrass, paint their faces or stomachs yellow, and wear a token (possibly made of otter skin) with the symbol of a snake or butterfly inscribed on it. In addition, they were never to lend an article of clothing to another person. If these interdictions were followed, pregnancy could be prevented. Schaeffer made notes about a woman who failed to follow the instructions given to her. Mrs. Phillip Arrowtop, after an extremely difficult delivery of her twins, approached Mrs. Chief Coward, who instructed her to paint her face and smudge her shawl and warned her never to lend an article of personal clothing to anyone. Mrs. Phillip Arrowtop broke these injunctions and, as a result, had two more children. Mrs. Chief Coward treated her again, and this time she did not transgress the prohibitions. She did not conceive again.[61]

These examples, although limited, point to a shared belief among northwestern Plains peoples that spiritual methods of contraception were effective. And they suggest that Aboriginal people relied on them because they worked. Historian Angus McLaren criticizes historians for failing to discuss "magic's" ability to influence fertility. Historians instead regard these methods as evidence that a culture does not possess contraceptive knowledge.[62] This assumption ignores the psychological impact these methods have on people. The term *birth control* does not necessarily apply solely to interrupting the biological process of conception (the sperm meeting the egg); it can also refer to a whole range of methods. Schaeffer, for example, noted that the Siksika used late weaning as a means to regulate and time births. Old Lady Bull Calf told him that "a mother would instruct her married daughter to let [her] body nurse until [the baby] stops of its own accord."[63] According to Old Lady Bull Calf, a woman should "nurse [her] baby as long as she desires, whenever the child wants another sibling she will cease."[64] Western science now acknowledges that breast-feeding reduces a woman's fertility.

Beverly Hungry Wolf relates a story told to her by her grandmothers regarding the spiritual powers that were used to prevent childbirth:

> The ones who had these powers would make up symbols of snakes or butterflies, which were considered powerful in child birth. These were given to women who wanted no children. They had to wear them all the time, next to their bodies. For instance, snakes were made from buckskin, stuffed, and worn like a belt. The stuffings were made of special materials, and the snake bodies were specially covered with beadwork and sacred paints. Often the women were instructed to stand over a smudge of special incense, so that the smoke could rise up to their bodies. They had to do this every night for as long as they wanted no more children.[65]

The use of visible markers to indicate a desire to limit fertility suggests that the onus or expectation for birth control did not fall solely on the shoulders of one of the participants: the markers were about informing *both* participants. Perhaps because birth control practices were relatively common knowledge in the community, there was a sense of shared responsibility – that is, both women and men were involved in these decisions. In a hunting and gathering community in which mobility was of paramount importance and resources were limited, responsibility for limiting the size of the community was shared by all and essential to societal well-being.

Ceremonial and spiritual forms of birth control were not the only methods practised by the Siksika. In the 1930s Goldfrank's informant Hilda told her: "Women take medicine to keep from having children. Many get it from a medicine woman. She knew of one woman who, when her period did not come, took a strong drink of pepper tea so as not to have kids – knows of no other kind of abortion. Women will go to a medicine woman for a brew when they are pregnant."[66]

An informant likewise provided Schaeffer with evidence that women used certain types of roots for abortion. This person also told him that abortifacients were considered a bad thing and equivalent to murder and that practitioners were not highly regarded.[67] Only two women were recorded by Schaeffer as possessing such knowledge: Mrs. Home Gun and Mrs. Chief Coward. This information was given to Schaeffer by a woman named Mrs. Pete Home Gun, who made it clear that she had refused any aid offered by these women.[68] Given that abortion was illegal or difficult to obtain in Canada until 1988, the evidence provided by Schaeffer's informants about such practices was mediated by contemporary debates surrounding abortion and birth control. In 1969 George First Rider revealed that a woman who did not want to get pregnant could drink a combination of three herbs: cut-leaf anemone, crooked stem, and wild liquorice.[69]

John Hellson and Morgan Gadd's work on Siksika plant use based on interviews in the 1970s records two ways in which birth control was practised. One method involved a special ceremonial bundle; the other was a herbal mixture that contained abortifacients. According to Hellson and Gadd, the anti-conception bundle was the property of a specific practitioner whose services could be purchased, whereas the herbal mixture was something a woman could use on her own.[70] Hellson and Gadd's informants recounted information consistent with that related by George First Rider, Schaeffer, Goldfrank, and Duvall, who each offered some evidence regarding the objects and materials that prevented conception. These items were otter skin wristlets with the design of a snake, yellow ochre, and some plant material.[71] Hellson and Gadd's informants indicated that the plant materials were the flowers and leaves of the new birch sucker *(Betula occidentalis)*, which were ingested if the bundle failed to prevent conception. Hellson and Gadd identified two other plants as abortifacients: *Anemone multifida* (crooked stem) and *Draba incerta* (yellowstone draba).[72] These researchers' field notes in conjunction with oral histories and ethnobotanical studies reveal that Aboriginal people relied on both medicinal plants and the spiritual to prevent conception.

The wealth of information about contraception and midwifery available in field notes from the 1930s is remarkable. Besides the social and legal taboos surrounding birth control, perhaps gender accounts for the failure of earlier ethnographers and anthropologists to publish about such practices. Unless Aboriginal women "invited them in," it was nearly impossible for anthropologists to gain access to certain sites of activity. Or maybe these earlier male observers did not consider methods of birth control and childbirth noteworthy. The presence of female researchers during the late 1930s provided the field of anthropology with a different perspective and opened the door to gendered sites of information that had long been closed to researchers. It is disappointing, then, that female anthropologists, even though they had access to the knowledge of Plains peoples about midwifery and birth control, chose not to publish any of it. Perhaps they, too, were worried about the legal ramifications of disseminating information about birth control. Hellson and Gadd did publish their information about Aboriginal birth control, but they did so in 1974, which had a different political and social environment.

Conclusion

Although they are but mere fragments, the above anecdotes show that Aboriginal midwives were active in their communities, made essential services available, relied on a repertoire of knowledge, stepped in when Western biomedicine failed to provide adequate services, and offered both immediate and long-term care to members of their communities.[73] None of these examples provide definitive or quantitative evidence regarding how prevalent Aboriginal midwifery practices were in the late nineteenth and early twentieth centuries. They do, however, indicate that these traditions remained valuable in Plains societies and contributed to the health and well-being of individuals and the community more generally.

What remains unclear is the extent to which Aboriginal therapeutic models remained a viable alternative in Aboriginal communities after the Second World War. The growing intrusion of Western health care services, the increasing formal and informal restrictions on traditional religious and medical practices, and the various methods implemented by the federal government to assimilate Aboriginal peoples made it very difficult for Aboriginal women healers to continue to openly provide their curative services. Joan Scott-Brown's study of the Nakoda in the 1970s suggests that medicine women remained important resources, that Aboriginal medicine remained a vital component of Aboriginal people's lives, and that healers were deeply respected individuals in the community and possessed the faith and trust of its members.[74]

Oral histories and the texts and unpublished papers of anthropologists who studied the peoples of southern Alberta reveal that, despite efforts by the churches and the state to replace Aboriginal medicine, the healing work of Aboriginal women persisted. Hospitals and residential schools run by the DIA reduced but did not erase the practice of midwifery among Aboriginal peoples. Taken in isolation, the anthropological evidence presented in Chapter 2 can be seen as unique or exceptional. When considered in conjunction with the evidence from Chapter 3 and the observations of anthropologists from the late 1930s, a persuasive pattern emerges: Aboriginal midwives formed long-lasting relationships with women in their communities by providing pre- and postnatal care and were able to offer women some relief from the pain of delivery. That there are similarities in the curative work of Aboriginal women over fifty years implies that the incidents recorded by ethnographers, anthropologists, and Euro-Canadian settlers were not unusual – indeed, they suggest that Aboriginal health care remained relevant to Aboriginal people long after the creation of reserves and the arrival of Western physicians, nurses, and hospitals.

Conclusion

In 1888 the Reverend E.F. Wilson, a missionary and amateur ethnographer, published an account of the Tsuu T'ina of southern Alberta in a *Report of the British Association for the Advancement of Science*. That account contains Wilson's observations about the history and culture of the Tsuu T'ina. His descriptions of Tsuu T'ina medical practices are of particular interest to this study. According to Wilson, the Tsuu T'ina "depend chiefly on magic and witchcraft for recovery from illness. There are about a dozen so-called 'medicine-men' in the camp, but most of them are *women*. Chief among them is an old squaw named 'Good Lodge.'"[1] Wilson dismissed the healing knowledge of the Tsuu T'ina in two ways. By referring to Aboriginal medicine as magic and witchcraft, he denied the existence of an extensive tradition of knowledge based on experience and practice. Furthermore, he repudiated medicine men by feminizing them; in other words, he considered Aboriginal medicine to be worthless because it was carried out by women. Wilson's derogatory comments draw attention to a relatively overlooked aspect of northwestern Plains peoples' cultural practices – the curative and caregiving work of women. Historians and anthropologists in recent years have done much to counteract the negative portrayal of Aboriginal women and Aboriginal healing and cultural practices. Even so, few scholars have systematically examined the gender-specific therapeutic roles played by Aboriginal women from the 1880s to the 1930s.

The buffalo hunter and the medicine man are two enduring symbols of northwestern Plains cultures. The currency of these masculine images reflects the fascination of generations of non-Aboriginal observers but does little to help us understand the complexity of Aboriginal cultures. This study addresses a significant and often overlooked aspect of northwestern Plains cultures by investigating the key roles that Siksika, Kainai, Piikuni, Tsuu T'ina, and Nakoda women played as healers and caregivers in the therapeutic regimes of Aboriginal peoples. Aboriginal women were vital to the health and well-being of their communities. In both Aboriginal and settler societies, women were responsible for specific curative skills and caregiving practices. This healing work in turn helped shape Western settlement and Aboriginal-white relations, and it served as a site of cultural resistance and conflict.

This study suggests that in northwestern Plains societies the gendered division of labour extended to curative knowledge and expertise. Aboriginal women in southern Alberta were responsible for the substantive and practical elements of health care, such as midwifery and medicinal plant use. Activities such as childbirth and the harvesting and preparation of wild plants often took place in private, female-centred space or in less visible spaces such as stands of trees. These activities were therefore harder to observe and less likely to be recorded. Even so, the published texts of ethnographers and anthropologists who observed northwestern Plains cultures in the late nineteenth and early twentieth centuries allow us a glimpse of women's work. When they are placed alongside other comparable materials, they allow a more complex picture of Aboriginal healing practices to emerge.

The arrival of Euro-Canadian settlers, especially women, in western Canada set the stage for new relationships between Aboriginal peoples and newcomers – relationships premised on healing and caregiving. White women, far from family and close female friends, relied on Aboriginal women for assistance during childbirth, for advice about medicinal plants and local resources, and for nursing care during illnesses and emergencies. During the early years of settlement, Aboriginal women played an important role in an informal network of healing and caregiving. Accounts of Aboriginal women providing midwifery or healing services to white settlers declined in number by the turn of the last century; however, white people's need for Aboriginal women's curative expertise did not end all at once. For some marginalized racial and ethnic groups and for people who lived in areas where there was little access to Western medicine, Aboriginal women's healing work remained a necessary alternative.

Yet notions of race and culture continued to strongly shape encounters among women. The movements of Aboriginal people were increasingly circumscribed as white settlers went about establishing a society premised on middle-class Euro-Canadian notions of respectability without considering the Aboriginal peoples who already occupied the land. Within this emerging white settler society, Aboriginal women were either invisible or perceived as a social and moral problem, especially in towns and cities. Aboriginal women might have gained entry to the private and domestic space of settlers, but they remained invisible. As historian Andrea Smith so appropriately writes, they were "a present absence."[2] In speeches, letters to family and friends, and newspaper articles, female settlers and missionaries lamented the lack of womanly companionship (effectively erasing Aboriginal women from the category of *women*) as well as their inadequate access to Western medicine – specifically, aid during childbirth. Aboriginal women entered the homes of Euro-Canadian women and touched white bodies, but their presence went unacknowledged. It is confusing and contradictory that the same people who relied on Aboriginal women's therapeutic skills appropriated Aboriginal land and denigrated their culture.

In contrast, the curative work that Euro-Canadian women performed, both for their own families and for Aboriginal people, received a great deal of applause and public attention and was characterized as either heroic pioneering maternalism or as a harbinger of civilization. The missionaries' wives and female missionaries who lived and worked in southern Alberta as early as the 1870s never publicly acknowledged their own participation in this informal network of healing. Euro-Canadian missionary women received assistance from Aboriginal women during childbirth and illnesses; in return, they provided Aboriginal people with medical help and nursing care at the mission house. Following the creation of reserves after 1877, the mission house became an important site for Aboriginal people to access medical help and nursing care. However, the therapeutic aid of Euro-Canadian women and missionaries' wives was accompanied by religious and domestic instruction and by the institutionalization of missionary medicine after the 1890s. This signalled the end of reciprocity, however unequal, between female missionaries and Aboriginal women.

Settlement on reserves during the 1880s and changing access to food resources led to starvation and ill health in many western Aboriginal communities. This taxed the resources and ability of missionaries' wives and female missionaries to treat Aboriginal people at the mission house and in residential schools. Concerned about the health of their potential converts, churches and their missionary organizations moved beyond the mission house to build Western-style health care institutions such as cottage hospitals, school infirmaries, and dispensaries. These facilities challenged Aboriginal women's healing and caregiving work. Western medicine became a standard by which Aboriginal motherhood was measured. Yet Aboriginal women continued to resist aspects of Western medicine, which was often not as effective as their own medicine, culturally irrelevant, or unaffordable. Midwifery was one field of practice in which missionary women and Department of Indian Affairs (DIA) medical officers had very little success. Not until the 1920s did Aboriginal women in growing numbers begin to use reserve hospitals for childbirth. And this development occurred only after residential schooling had interrupted the intergenerational transmission of midwifery knowledge and after DIA hospitals had begun to meet Aboriginal people's expectations by allowing children to remain with their mothers during confinement.

In the early twentieth century, trained nurses were in short supply, especially in the Prairie West. As a result, church-run facilities were operated mainly by women who had acquired their knowledge and nursing skill through experience and practice. The place of Euro-Canadian women in this developing system was significant, for it was they who lived full-time at reserves and who carried out the bulk of curative and nursing work. Mission societies, and later the DIA, relied on the affordable labour of female health care personnel, who could be paid less than doctors and were easier to recruit. Under this system, female health workers enjoyed greater autonomy in their work. After 1920 the issues of training and appropriate skills brought female health workers – including the Sisters of Charity – under fire. Experienced women who had developed relationships with the communities in which they worked were replaced by lay public health nurses who did not live in reserve communities or speak Aboriginal languages. This development fundamentally altered the patient-practitioner relationship.

The standard of living for Aboriginal people improved very little during the early twentieth century. Infectious diseases associated with poverty and poor living conditions – such as tuberculosis and trachoma – replaced smallpox as the greatest threats to health. The ill health of Aboriginal people remained rooted in inadequate housing, crowded living conditions, poor and insufficient food, and scant clothing. To the DIA's chagrin, and despite the department's best efforts, expenditures for Aboriginal medical care continued to rise. After 1915, to stem growing medical costs, the DIA began taking over the health system that the church missions had established. By 1927, when Indian Health Services (IHS) was formally created, Western health care was deeply entrenched in Treaty 7 communities. The

DIA would rely until after the Second World War on the piecemeal system of cottage hospitals, school infirmaries, and dispensaries that had been founded by the churches and staffed by female workers. After 1920 the Euro-Canadian women employed by the DIA were expected to possess formal nursing credentials.

The federal government, through the IHS, made public health instruction and the prevention of contagious diseases its primary objectives. A system of travelling public health nurses was created to provide Aboriginal women with instruction in domestic hygiene and child care. In reserve communities that had especially poor health conditions and in which the infant mortality rate remained high, the department assigned permanent public health nurses. The nurses' tasks included tracking expectant mothers, attending childbirths, and offering postnatal care and instruction. The bodies of Aboriginal women, the medical choices they made, and their mothering practices became sites of cultural difference and colonization during the 1920s.

Despite the presence of DIA medical facilities and the attendance of graduate and public health nurses, nursing sisters, and female attendants, the therapeutic work of Aboriginal women persisted well into the twentieth century. Oral histories and the field notes of anthropologists who conducted fieldwork in southern Alberta during the late 1930s suggest that women's healing and caregiving labour remained relevant to Aboriginal communities. Instead of replacing Aboriginal medicine, biomedicine and medical institutions coexisted with Aboriginal models of health and healing. The medical choices Aboriginal people made were based on proven effectiveness and the perceived origins of the disease at hand. In particular, the obstetrical knowledge of Aboriginal midwives and the presence of experienced female family members endured in Aboriginal communities, despite the state's best efforts to undermine and criminalize such practices. That Aboriginal women continued to make these services available in the face of strong campaigns against them is indicative of their cultural strength and survival.

Aboriginal peoples adapted to Western medicine and incorporated elements of it into their existing cultural strategies. All the while, Aboriginal medicine encountered enormous opposition from the DIA. Aboriginal health practitioners were denigrated and characterized as harmful to their communities. Meanwhile, the residential schools interfered with the transmission of curative knowledge and skills. The relative success of Aboriginal midwives and the inability of certain DIA institutions to care for maternity cases until the 1920s made it unlikely that Aboriginal women would use DIA hospitals for childbirth. By the end of the period under study, however, advances in asepsis, anaesthetics, and surgical techniques had changed the choices Aboriginal women made about birth attendants and location. Improvements in Western medicine enhanced women's chances of surviving childbirth in demonstrable ways.

By tracing the patterns of women's healing and caregiving work in Aboriginal communities, this study highlights overlooked facets of western settlement. First, Aboriginal women possessed knowledge and proficiency in midwifery and the healing properties of local plants. This expertise remained an important cultural and economic resource for Treaty 7 communities during the demographic and economic crisis that developed between the 1880s and the 1930s. This study shows that Aboriginal curative knowledge persisted among the people of the northwestern Plains, it documents its gender-specific dimensions, and it shows how gender operated in particular forms of cultural resistance and change.

Second, this study explores the health care work performed by Euro-Canadian women in Treaty 7 communities during the late nineteenth and early twentieth centuries. It investigates the nursing work carried out by women in Catholic congregations and Protestant missions and by graduate nurses employed by the DIA and reveals that missionary organizations and government agencies relied on women's labour. The labour of female nursing personnel was more readily available and less expensive than that of male doctors. By documenting the health care work undertaken by nurses, this study extends knowledge of colonial health care in Canada, which to date is concentrated on male doctors and government officials.

Indeed, the evidence of women's work laid out here highlights the often overlooked role played by missionary organizations. Existing literature on the creation of the DIA health system fails to note the close links between the state and the church missions. The Catholic orders and Protestant missions did much to shape Western medical services on Treaty 7 reserves. They also influenced a reluctant federal government to fund institutions and personnel. Yet, at the same time, mission hospitals and school infirmaries kept Aboriginal children in residential schools when they were sick or injured instead of sending them home. The healing work of Euro-Canadian women, trained or not, remained central to this system.

Third and finally, this study reveals that health care in southern Alberta created spaces – however brief and unequal – where women from vastly different cultures could meet. This contact sometimes occurred in the homes of Aboriginal people, but most often it was in the homes of Euro-Canadian settlers or at the mission house, where women shared midwifery, botanical, and medical skills. Cultures were brought into contact through childbirth and family illnesses. The basis of these encounters was women's shared responsibilities for household tasks and child care. In some instances, the women of southern Alberta recognized the common bond of gender — for example, when they delivered babies, shared valuable economic skills, or even (occasionally) told DIA officials that local water supplies were inadequate.

Ideas about Aboriginal peoples' racial inferiority survived, however, even in the face of settlers' dependence on Aboriginal women. Contact more often reinforced the power relations of colonialism as Euro-Canadian women used their intimate relationships with Aboriginal women to undermine Aboriginal peoples' cultural practices. As women, the health workers hired by the DIA and the mission societies gained access to gendered sites of domestic production and reproduction. Their male counterparts did not. When white women entered the homes of Aboriginal women, they tried to teach them Euro-Canadian values and ideas of domesticity and child care. Euro-Canadian women played active and significant roles in colonial regimes. The gendered domestic work of health care was a location of colonial encounter that deserves greater analysis today.

Notes

Introduction

1 The term *nursing care* is used to refer to the bedside care of a patient, which involves personal care and hygiene, feeding, and therapeutic functions.
2 Sherry Smith, *Reimagining Indians: Native Americans through Anglo Eyes, 1880-1940* (New York: Oxford University Press, 2000), 3.
3 During the late nineteenth century, the term *graduate nurse* came into use to distinguish those women who had completed a three-year apprenticeship in nursing at hospital-training schools from those women who had not. For further information, see Kathryn McPherson, *Bedside Matters: The Transformation of Canadian Nursing, 1900-1990* (Don Mills, ON: Oxford University Press, 1996).
4 Linda Gordon, "Internal Colonialism and Gender," in *Haunted by Empire: Geographies of Intimacy in North American History*, ed. Ann Laura Stoler (Durham, NC: Duke University Press, 2006), 429-31.
5 For a discussion of mission work and the establishment of a "state of colonialism," see Jean Comaroff, *Body of Power, Spirit of Resistance: The Culture and History of a South African People* (Chicago: University of Chicago Press, 1985); and Jean Comaroff and John Comaroff, eds., *Civil Society and the Political Imagination in Africa: Critical Perspectives* (Chicago: University of Chicago Press, 1999).
6 Maureen Lux, *Medicine That Walks: Disease, Medicine, and Canadian Plains Native People, 1880-1940* (Toronto: University of Toronto Press, 2001), and Mary-Ellen Kelm, *Colonizing Bodies: Aboriginal Health and Healing in British Columbia, 1900-1950* (Vancouver: UBC Press, 1998).
7 Philippa Levine, *Prostitution, Race, and Politics: Policing Venereal Disease in the British Empire* (New York: Routledge, 2003), 201-7.
8 Nayan Shah, "Cleansing Motherhood: Hygiene and the Culture of Domesticity in San Francisco's Chinatown, 1875-1900," in *Gender, Sexuality, and Colonial Modernities*, ed. Antoinette Burton (London: Routledge, 1999), 25.

9 Ann Laura Stoler, "Tense and Tender Ties: The Politics of Comparison in North American History and (Post) Colonial Studies," in *Haunted by Empire: Geographies of Intimacy in North American History*, ed. Ann Laura Stoler (Durham, NC: Duke University Press, 2006), 35-36. See also Anne McClintock, "No Longer in a Future Heaven: Gender, Race, and Nationalism," in *Dangerous Liaisons: Gender, Nation, and Postcolonial Perspectives*, ed. Anne McClintock, Aamir Rashid Mufti, and Ella Shohat (Minneapolis: University of Minnesota Press, 1997), 89-113.
10 Catherine Hall, "Commentary," in *Haunted by Empire*, ed. Stoler, 457.
11 Ann Laura Stoler, *Carnal Knowledge and Imperial Power: Race and the Intimate in Colonial Rule* (Berkeley: University of California Press, 2002), 205-6.
12 Anne McClintock, *Imperial Leather: Race, Gender, and Sexuality in the Colonial Contest* (New York: Routledge, 1995), 6.
13 Katie Pickles and Myra Rutherdale, "Introduction," in *Contact Zones: Aboriginal and Settler Women in Canada's Colonial Past*, ed. Pickles and Rutherdale (Vancouver: UBC Press, 2005), 1.
14 Nancy Pagh, *At Home Afloat: Women on the Waters of the Pacific Northwest* (Calgary: University of Calgary Press, 2001), 107-11. See also Dianne Newell, "Belonging – Out of Place: Women's Travelling Stories from the Western Edge," in *Contact Zones*, ed. Pickles and Rutherdale, 246-71.
15 Myra Rutherdale, *Women and the White Man's God: Gender and Race in the Canadian Mission Field* (Vancouver: UBC Press, 2002), 42-49.
16 Barbara Kelcy, *Alone in Silence: European Women in the Canadian North before 1940* (Montreal/Kingston: McGill-Queen's University Press, 2001), 130-41.
17 Sarah Carter, "First Nations Women and Colonization on the Canadian Prairies, 1870s-1920s," in *Rethinking Canada: The Promise of Women's History*, ed. Veronica Strong-Boag, Mona Gleason, and Adele Perry, 4th ed. (Don Mills, ON: Oxford University Press, 2002), 142.
18 Adele Perry, *On the Edge of Empire: Gender, Race, and the Making of British Columbia, 1849-1871* (Toronto: University of Toronto Press, 2001), 48-75.
19 Similar arguments are made about Aboriginal women in Victoria, BC. Jean Barman, "Aboriginal Women on the Streets of Victoria: Rethinking Transgressive Sexuality during the Colonial Encounter," in *Contact Zones*, ed. Pickles and Rutherdale, 205-27.
20 Linda McDowell, *Gender, Identity, and Place: Understanding Feminist Geographies* (Minneapolis: University of Minnesota Press, 1999), 72.
21 The term *Indian* is outdated, inappropriate, and historically inaccurate. I use it only in quotations from primary sources and in reference to legal and constitutive matters. There are three legal categories of Indians in Canada: Status Indians (individuals who are registered with the federal government according to criteria outlined in the Indian Act); Non-Status Indians (individuals who are members of a First Nation but whom the federal government does not recognize as Indians according to criteria laid out in the Indian Act); and Treaty Indians (individuals who are Status Indians and recognized members of a First Nation that signed a treaty with the Crown). Legislation aimed exclusively at Aboriginal women complicates the issue of identity and terminology further; Section 6 of the 1869 Indian Act stipulated that an Aboriginal woman who married a non-Aboriginal man ceased to be an Indian. This disenfranchisement also applied to band membership. If a woman married an individual from another tribe or band, she, in the eyes of the government, severed ties

to and lost membership in her natal band. For further information regarding the Indian Act and Aboriginal women, see Kathleen Jamieson, *Indian Women and the Law in Canada: Citizens Minus* (Ottawa: Advisory Council on the Status of Women, 1978).

22 The term *First Nations* is used to replace the word *band* or *tribe* in the naming of communities. Indian and Northern Affairs Canada, Communications Branch, "Words First: An Evolving Terminology Relating to Aboriginal Peoples in Canada," Collections Canada, October 2002, http://www.collectionscanada.gc.ca/webarchives/20071115071229/http://www.ainc-inac.gc.ca/pr/pub/wf/pdf_e.html.

23 Elizabeth Vibert, "Real Men Hunt Buffalo: Masculinity, Race, and Class in British Fur Traders' Narratives," in *Gender and History in Canada,* ed. Joy Parr and Mark Rosenfeld (Mississauga, ON: Copp Clark, 1996), 51.

24 Franz Boas was born and educated in Germany, where he earned a doctorate in physics. In the early 1990s, he travelled to the United States, where he worked for the Bureau of Ethnology until his appointment to Columbia University in 1896.

25 Paul Erickson and Liam Murphy, *A History of Anthropological Theory,* 2nd ed. (Peterborough, ON: Broadview Press, 2003), 73-76.

26 William Taylor, Foreword to *The Indians of Canada,* by Diamond Jenness (Toronto: University of Toronto Press, 1977), v.

Chapter 1: Niitsitapi

1 David McCrady, *Living with Strangers: The Nineteenth-Century Sioux and the Canadian-American Borderlands* (Lincoln: University of Nebraska Press, 2006).

2 John Ewers, *The Blackfeet: Raiders on the Northwestern Plains* (Norman: University of Oklahoma Press, 1958), 6-7.

3 Colin Taylor and Hugh Dempsey, *With Eagle Tail: Arnold Lupson and Thirty Years among the Sarcee, Blackfoot, and Stoney Indians on the North American Plains* (New York: Salamander, 1999), 52. Aboriginal people have their own creation stories, which remain vital and relevant to their communities.

4 Hugh Dempsey, "The Blackfoot Indians," in *Native Peoples: The Canadian Experience,* ed. R. Bruce Morrison and C. Roderick Wilson, 2nd ed. (Toronto: McClelland and Stewart, 1995), 381.

5 Elizabeth Churchill, "Tsuu T'ina: A History of a First Nations Community, 1890-1940" (PhD diss., University of Calgary, 2000), 2.

6 Rev. E.F. Wilson, "Report on the Sarcee Indians," *Report of the British Association for the Advancement of Science* 58 (1888): 243. See also Theodore Binnema, *Common and Contested Ground: A Human and Environmental History of the Northwestern Plains* (Norman: University of Okalahoma Press, 2001), 83.

7 Diamond Jenness, *The Sarcee Indians of Alberta* (Ottawa: National Museum of Canada, 1938), 8-9.

8 Binnema, *Common and Contested Ground,* 116-17; Alan McMillan, *Native Peoples and Cultures of Canada* (Toronto: Douglas and McIntyre, 1990), 154.

9 Taylor, *With Eagle Tail,* 92.

10 Ibid., 95.

11 David Jones, *Empire of Dust: Settling and Abandoning the Prairie Dry Belt* (Edmonton: University of Alberta Press, 1987), 42-44.

12 Dempsey, "The Blackfoot Indians," 384.
13 Mary Melainey and Barbara Sherriff, "Adjusting Our Perceptions: Historical and Archaeological Evidence of Winter on the Plains of Western Canada," *Plains Anthropologist* 41, 158 (1996): 333-57.
14 Sarah Carter, *Aboriginal People and Colonizers of Western Canada to 1900* (Toronto: University of Toronto Press, 1999), 24-25.
15 Andrew Isenberg, *The Destruction of the Buffalo* (Cambridge: Cambridge University Press, 2000), 75-80. See also Carter, *Aboriginal People and Colonizers*, 24-25.
16 Sarah Carter, "First Nations Women and Colonization on the Canadian Prairies, 1870s-1920s," in *Rethinking Canada: The Promise of Women's History*, ed. Veronica Strong-Boag, Mona Gleason, and Adele Perry (Don Mills, ON: Oxford University Press, 2002), 137-47.
17 Joan Jensen, *Calling This Place Home: Women on the Wisconsin Frontier, 1850-1925* (Minneapolis: Minnesota Historical Society Press, 2006), 100-7.
18 Elman Service, *The Hunters* (New Jersey: Prentice-Hall, 1966), 7-8.
19 Alice Kehoe, "How the Ancient Peigans Lived," *Research in Economic Anthropology* 14 (1993): 87-105.
20 Reg Crowshoe and Sybille Manneschmidt, *Akak'stiman: A Blackfoot Framework for Decision-Making and Mediation Processes* (Calgary: University of Calgary Press, 2001), 15.
21 Tribes are similar to bands in that they are a collection of individual nuclear families combined to form larger units. Tribes are, however, larger and more complex than bands. The difference lies in the organization of pan-tribal associations "because they cross-cut the residential segments of the society, such as households and bands and unite social and politically." Elman Service, *Profiles in Ethnology*, 3rd ed. (New York: Harper and Row, 1978), 4-6.
22 Adolf Hungry Wolf, *The Blackfoot Papers – Volume One: Pikunni History and Culture* (Skookumchuck, BC: Good Medicine Cultural Foundation, 2006), 65.
23 Ibid.
24 Crowshoe and Manneschmidt, *Akak'stiman*, 16.
25 Service defines a sodality as a "nonresidential association that has some corporate functions or purposes." Elman Service, *Primitive Social Organization: An Evolutionary Perspective* (New York: Random House, 1962), 21.
26 Treaty 7 Elders and Tribal Council et al., *The True Spirit and Original Intent of Treaty 7* (Montreal/Kingston: McGill-Queen's University Press, 1996), 83.
27 Dempsey, "The Blackfoot Indians," 391.
28 Crowshoe, *Akak'stiman*, 18.
29 Dempsey, "The Blackfoot Indians," 390.
30 Clark Wissler and D.C. Duvall, *Mythology of the Blackfoot Indians* (Lincoln: University of Nebraska Press, 1995 [1908]), 74-90. See also Gerald Mohatt and Joseph Eagle Elk, *The Price of a Gift: A Lakota Healer's Story* (Lincoln: University of Nebraska Press, 2000), 130-32.
31 Clark Wissler, "The Sun Dance of the Blackfoot Indians," in *A Blackfoot Source Book: Papers by Clark Wissler*, ed. David Hurst Thomas (New York: Garland, 1986), 229-30.
32 Crowshoe, *Akak'stiman*, 21.
33 The Natoas bundle comprises the Holy Woman's headdress, a turnip digger, and an elk hide robe.
34 Wissler, "The Sun Dance of the Blackfoot Indians," 229.
35 Joan Scott-Brown, "Stoney Ethnobotany: An Indication of Cultural Change amongst Stoney Women of Morley, Alberta" (master's thesis, University of Calgary, 1977), 148-54.

36 Beatrice Medicine, "Warrior Women: Sex Role Alternatives for Plains Indian Women," in *The Hidden Half: Studies of Plains Indian Women*, ed. Patricia Albers and Beatrice Medicine (Lanham, MD: University Press of America, 1983), 267-80.
37 The Blackfoot Gallery Committee, *Nitsitapiisinni: The Story of the Blackfoot People* (Toronto: Key Porter, 2001), 26.
38 Ewers, *The Blackfeet*, 86. See also McMillan, *Native Peoples and Cultures of Canada*, 44.
39 John Ewers, *The Blackfeet*, 86.
40 Ibid., 84.
41 Elizabeth Vibert, "Real Men Hunt Buffalo: Masculinity, Race, and Class in British Fur Traders' Narratives," in *Gender and History in Canada*, ed. Joy Parr and Mark Rosenfeld (Mississauga, ON: Copp Clark, 1996).
42 Carter, "First Nations Women and Colonization," 138.
43 Carter, *Aboriginal People and Colonizers*, 90.
44 Oscar Lewis, "Manly-Hearted Women among the North Peigan," *American Anthropologist*, n.s., 43, 2 (1941): 175.
45 For examples of diverse forms of social organization, see Sarah Carter, *The Importance of Being Monogamous: Marriage and Nation Building in Western Canada to 1915* (Edmonton: Athabasca University Press/University of Alberta Press, 2008); and Evelyn Blackwood, *Female Desires: Same-Sex Relations and Transgender Practices across Cultures* (New York: Columbia University Press, 1999).
46 Evelyn Blackwood, "Sexuality and Gender in Certain Native American Tribes: The Case of Cross-Gender Females," *Signs* 10, 11 (1984): 27-42.
47 Alan Klein, "The Political-Economy of Gender: A Nineteenth-Century Plains Indian Case Study," in *The Hidden Half: Studies of Plains Indian Women*, ed. Patricia Albers and Beatrice Medicine (Lanham, MD: University Press of America, 1983), 143-73.
48 For an explanation of the term *cultural florescence*, see Bruce Trigger, "The French Presence in Huronia: The Structure of Franco-Huron Relations in the First Half of the 17th-Century," in *Readings in Canadian History: Pre-Confederation*, ed. Douglas Francis and Donald Smith, 6th ed. (Toronto: Nelson Thompson, 2002), 21-47.
49 For examples of the debate regarding the impact of the horse on northwestern Plains cultures, see John Ewers, *The Horse in Blackfeet Indian Culture: With Comparative Material from Other Western Tribes* (Washington, DC: Smithsonian Institution Press, 1955); Frank Gilbert Roe, *The Indian and the Horse* (Norman: University of Oklahoma Press, 1955); Demitri Shimkin, "The Introduction of the Horse," in *Handbook of North American Indians*, vol. 11, ed. Warren D'Azevedo (Washington, DC: Smithsonian Institution Press, 1986), 517-24.
50 Isenberg, *The Destruction of the Bison*, 92.
51 Frank Raymond Secoy, *Changing Military Patterns of the Great Plains* (New York: J.J. Augustin, 1953), 52.
52 Dempsey, "The Blackfoot Indians," 397.
53 Ibid., 405. For a debate regarding the destruction of the buffalo, see David Smits, "The Frontier Army and the Destruction of the Buffalo, 1865-1883," in *Uncommon Ground: Rethinking the Human Place in Nature*, ed. William Cronon (New York: Norton, 1995), 171-85; Dan Flores, "Bison Ecology and Bison Diplomacy: The Southern Plains from 1800 to 1850," *Journal of American History* 78, 2 (1991): 465-85; William Dobak, "Killing the Canadian Buffalo, 1821-1881," *Western Historical Quarterly* 27 (Spring 1996): 33-52.

54 Irene Spry, *The Palliser Expedition: An Account of John Palliser's British North American Expedition, 1857-1860* (Toronto: Macmillan, 1963), 60; Dobak, "Killing the Canadian Buffalo."
55 Linea Sundstrom, "Smallpox Used Them Up: References to Epidemic Disease in Northern Plains Winter Counts, 1714-1920," *Ethnohistory* 44, 2 (1997): 308. Winter counts are Aboriginal histories or calendars in which events are recorded with one picture for each year.
56 Jody Decker, "Tracing Historical Diffusion Patterns: The Case of the 1780-82 Smallpox Epidemic among the Indians of Western Canada," *Native Studies Review* 4, 1-2 (1988): 21.
57 Jody Decker, "Country Distempers: Deciphering Disease and Illness in Rupert's Land before 1870," in *Reading beyond Words: Contexts for Native History,* ed. Jennifer Brown and Elizabeth Vibert (Peterborough, ON: Broadview Press, 1998), 173. Paul Kelton describes the ways that southeastern Aboriginal peoples incorporated quarantine practices into their existing health care strategies in the eighteenth century. See Kelton, "Avoiding the Smallpox Spirits: Colonial Epidemics and Southeastern Indian Survival," *Ethnohistory* 51, 1 (2004): 45-71. Naomi Rogers, in *Dirt and Disease: Polio Before FDR* (New Brunswick, NJ: Rutgers University Press, 1992), makes a similar argument for North American society more generally. She argues that despite the introduction of germ theory and scientific medicine, ideas of disease causation remained deeply rooted in nineteenth-century beliefs.
58 John C. Hellson and Morgan Gadd, *Ethnobotany of the Blackfoot Indians* (Ottawa: National Museums of Canada, 1974), 74.
59 Canada, *Annual Report of the Department of Indian Affairs for the Year Ended June 30, 1899* (Ottawa: Queen's Printer, 1900), 132-33, 124, 125.
60 Ibid., 124.
61 Hugh Dempsey, *Indian Tribes of Alberta* (Calgary: Glenbow-Alberta Institute, 1978), 22.
62 Canada, *Annual Report of the Department of Indian Affairs for the Year Ended June 30, 1892* (Ottawa: Queen's Printer, 1893), 180; Canada, *Annual Report of the Department of Indian Affairs for the Year Ended June 30, 1891* (Ottawa: Queen's Printer, 1892), 59.
63 Canada, *Annual Report of the Department of Indian Affairs for the Year Ended June 30, 1898* (Ottawa: Queen's Printer, 1899), 168.
64 Ibid.
65 Ibid.
66 Patricia Wood, "Pressured from All Sides: The February 1913 Surrender of the Northeast Corner of the Tsuu T'ina Nation, *Journal of Historical Geography* 30, 1 (2004): 112.
67 Canada, *Annual Report of the Department of Indian Affairs for the Year Ended June 30, 1896* (Ottawa: Queen's Printer, 1897), 202.
68 Ibid.
69 Canada, *Annual Report (1892),* 179.
70 Sheila McManus, *The Line Which Separates: Race, Gender, and the Making of the Alberta-Montana Borderlands* (Lincoln: University of Nebraska Press, 2005), 67.
71 Carter, *Aboriginal People and Colonizers,* 95-96.
72 Howard Palmer and Tamara Palmer, *Alberta: A New History* (Edmonton: Hurtig, 1990), 107-9.
73 Ibid., 107-8.
74 John Tobias, "Protection, Civilization, Assimilation: An Outline History of Canada's Indian Policy," in *As Long as the Sun Shines and Water Flows: A Reader in Canadian Native Studies,* ed. Ian Getty and Antoine Lussier (Vancouver: UBC Press, 1983), 44.

75 Ibid., 46-49. See, for example, *An Act to further amend "The Indian Act, 1880,"* SC 1884 (47 Vict.), c. 27, s.3; *An Act to Further Amend the Indian Act,* SC 1895, c. 35, s. 3.
76 Douglas Leighton, "A Victorian Civil Servant at Work: Lawrence Vankoughnet and the Canadian Indian Department, 1874-1893," in *As Long as the Sun Shines and Water Flows,* ed. Getty and Lussier, 108-10.
77 Ewers, *The Blackfeet,* 294.
78 George Bird Grinnell, *Blackfoot Lodge Tales: The Story of a Prairie People* (Lincoln: University of Nebraska Press, 1962 [1892]), 289.
79 Hana Samek, *The Blackfoot Confederacy, 1880-1920: A Comparative Study of Canada and United States Indian Policy* (Albuquerque: University of New Mexico Press, 1987), 45.
80 For a detailed discussion, see Maureen Lux, *Medicine That Walks: Disease, Medicine, and Canadian Plains Native People, 1880-1940* (Toronto: University of Toronto Press, 2001), 20-70.
81 See the Introduction.
82 Report, Inspector McGibbon, November 1897, Library and Archives Canada (LAC), RG 10, Department of Indian Affairs, vol. 381, file 54, p. 550.
83 Hugh Dempsey, "One Hundred Years of Treaty Seven," in *One Century Later: Western Canadian Reserve Indians since Treaty 7,* ed. Ian Getty and Donald Smith (Vancouver: UBC Press, 1978), 28.
84 Canada, *Annual Reports of the Department of Indian Affairs for the Years Ended June 30, 1881-1918.*
85 Dr. Bryce to Wilfred Laurier, December 5, 1905, LAC, Wilfred Laurier Papers, vol. 291, file 104061-65; Megan Sproule-Jones, "Crusading for the Forgotten: Dr. Peter Bryce, Public Health, and Prairie Native Residential Schools," *Canadian Bulletin of Medical History/Bulletin canadien d'histoire* 13, 2 (1996): 204.
86 Gerald Friesen, *The Canadian Prairies: A History* (Toronto: University of Toronto Press, 1987), 236-41; Canada, *Annual Report of the Department of Indian Affairs for the Year Ended June 30, 1884* (Ottawa: Queen's Printer, 1885), 87.
87 Lux, *Medicine that Walks,* 65.
88 One of the first works to document the federal government's failure to fulfill treaty promises is Sarah Carter, *Lost Harvests: Prairie Indian Reserve Farmers and Government Policy* (Montreal/Kingston: McGill-Queen's University Press, 1990). For a more recent work, see Hugh Shewell, *Enough to Keep Them Alive: Indian Welfare in Canada, 1873 to 1965* (Toronto: University of Toronto Press, 2004).
89 Michael Lee McIntyre, "Sarcee Demography, 1880-1925" (master's thesis, University of Calgary, 1975), 35.
90 Lux, *Medicine That Walks,* 201.
91 Canada, *Annual Report of the Department of Indian Affairs for the Year Ended June 30, 1933* (Ottawa: King's Printer, 1933), 12-13.
92 For an overview of how historians have emphasized the relationship between standard of living and health, see Judith Leavitt and Ronald Numbers, "Sickness and Health in America: An Overview," in *Sickness and Health in America,* ed. Judith Leavitt and Ronald Numbers (Madison: University of Wisconsin Press, 1997), 3-10. See also Nancy Tomes, "The Private Side of Public Health: Sanitary Science, Domestic Hygiene, and the Germ Theory, 1870-1900," in *Sickness and Health in America,* ed. Leavitt and Numbers, 506-28.
93 Herbert Brown Ames, *The City Below the Hill* (Toronto: University of Toronto Press, 1972 [1897]), 80-81.

94 Lux, *Medicine That Walks.*
95 James B. Waldram, D. Ann Herring, and T. Kue Young, *Aboriginal Health in Canada: Historical, Cultural, and Epidemiological Perspectives,* 2nd ed. (Toronto: University of Toronto Press, 2006), 181-86. See also Lux, *Medicine That Walks,* 140.
96 Sproule-Jones, "Crusading for the Forgotten," 200.

Chapter 2: Setting the Stage

1 Daniel Francis, *The Imaginary Indian: The Image of the Indian in Canadian Culture* (Vancouver: Arsenal Pulp Press, 1992), 16-60.
2 Walter McClintock, *The Old North Trail: Life, Legends, and Religion of the Blackfoot Indians* (Lincoln: University of Nebraska Press, 1999 [1910], 104, 153.
3 Sherry Smith, *Reimagining Indians: Native Americans through Anglo Eyes, 1880-1940* (New York: Oxford University Press, 2000), 4-5.
4 Ibid., 59-66.
5 Grinnell, a Yale graduate, was a naturalist and editor of the magazine *Field and Stream.* Although he also wrote about the Cheyenne and Pawnee, his best-known work is *Blackfoot Lodge Tales: The Story of a Prairie People.* His first contact with the Blackfeet was precipitated by correspondence with James Willard Schultz, who contacted Grinnell during the winter of 1883-84 in an effort to secure aid from the United States government for starving Blackfeet in Montana. In 1885 Grinnell visited Montana to study the Blackfeet. He was adopted into the tribe, named Pinutoyi Istsimokan (or Fisher Hat), and made an honorary chief.
6 James Willard Schultz, a friend and frequent correspondent of Grinnell, was educated at Peekskill Military Academy. In 1877 he travelled west to hunt buffalo and work as a fur trader. He married a Piikani named Fine Shield Woman, from whom he learned the Blackfoot language. He remained in Montana until the death of Fine Shield Woman in 1902. With the encouragement and financial support of Grinnell, he wrote about his life among the Blackfeet. His first book, *My Life as an Indian,* originally published as a magazine series by *Field and Stream,* was republished by Doubleday in 1907.
7 John Maclean was an ordained Methodist minister who served as a missionary at the Blood Reserve in southern Alberta from 1880 to 1889. After retiring from the mission field in 1889, he devoted much of his time to writing books and speaking on lecture tours about Native North Americans. In 1892 he published his first book, *Indians of Canada: Their Manners and Customs.* This was followed in 1896 by his best-known work, *Canadian Savage Folk.*
8 The final ethnographer is Walter McClintock. McClintock was born in Pittsburgh, Pennsylvania, in 1870. He graduated in 1891 from Yale. After working in his parents' carpet business for five years, he joined a government expedition to the northern Rockies. The expedition's goal was to gather data for a forest reserve policy for federal land. During the journey he became acquainted with two of the guides, Billy Jackson and Jack Monroe. Jackson and Munroe had also served as guides for George Bird Grinnell in 1885. Jackson invited McClintock to his home in Cutbank Creek, where McClintock began collecting Blackfeet stories. During his visit he was adopted by Mad Wolf and given a Blackfoot name, A-pe-ech eken (White Weasel). *The Old North Trail* was published in 1910.
9 Darrell Robes Kipp, Introduction to *Blackfeet Tales of Glacier National Park,* by James W. Schultz (Helena, MO: Riverbend, 2002 [1916]), vii-ix.

10 Carol Higham, "Saviors and Scientists: North American Protestant Missionaries and the Development of Anthropology," *Pacific Historical Review* 72, 4 (2003): 531. See also Mary Louise Pratt, *Imperial Eyes: Travel Writing and Transculturation* (London: Routledge, 1992).
11 Alice Kehoe, Introduction to *Mythology of the Blackfoot Indians,* by Clark Wissler and D.C. Duvall (Lincoln: University of Nebraska Press, 1995 [1908]), v.
12 Ibid., vi.
13 Ibid., vii.
14 Ibid., x.
15 For a similar situation in a different cultural context, see Judy Thompson, *Recording Their Story: James and the Tahltan* (Vancouver: Douglas and McIntyre, 2007).
16 John Maclean, "Blackfoot Medical Priesthood," *Medicine Hat News,* October 21, 1909.
17 McClintock, *The Old North Trail,* 169.
18 Ibid.
19 George Bird Grinnell, *Blackfoot Lodge Tales: The Story of a Prairie People* (Lincoln: University of Nebraska Press, 1962 [1892]), 284.
20 McClintock, *The Old North Trail,* 168-69; Grinnell, *Blackfoot Lodge Tales,* 284.
21 McClintock, *The Old North Trail,* 168-69. See also John Maclean, *Canadian Savage Folk: The Native Tribes of Canada* (Toronto: William Briggs, 1896), 201-6.
22 Rufus Goodstriker, Kainai elder, February 14, 1983, First Nations University of Canada (FNUC), Indian History Film Projects (IHFP), IH 007.
23 McClintock, *The Old North Trail,* 253. For further examples, see Clark Wissler, *Social Organization and Ritualistic Ceremonies of the Blackfoot Indians* (New York: AMS, 1912), 82, 84.
24 Pliny Earle Goddard, "Sarsi Texts," *University of California Publications in American Archaeology and Ethnology* 11, 3 (1915): 224-45. Goddard describes the acquisition of several different types of medicines, all of which follow the same prescriptive format.
25 McClintock, *The Old North Trail,* 142.
26 Michael Angel, *Preserving the Sacred: Historical Perspectives on the Ojibwa Midewiwin* (Winnipeg: University of Manitoba Press, 2002), 67.
27 James Waldram, D. Ann Herring, and T. Kue Young, *Aboriginal Health in Canada: Historical, Cultural, and Epidemiological Perspectives,* 2nd ed. (Toronto: University of Toronto Press, 2006), 99-100.
28 Grinnell, *Blackfoot Lodge Tales,* 281, 284.
29 James Schultz, *Blackfeet Tales of Glacier National Park* (Helena, MO: Riverbend Publishing, 2002 [1916]), 199.
30 McClintock, *The Old North Trail,* 364, 524-31.
31 Sandra Leslie Peacock, "Piikani Ethnobotany: Traditional Plant Knowledge of the Piikani Peoples of the Northwestern Plains" (master's thesis, University of Calgary, 1992), 24.
32 McClintock, *The Old North Trail,* 235-36.
33 Ibid., 364.
34 Rufus Goodstriker, Kainai elder, February 14, 1983.
35 Marion Carrier, Cree elder, July 30, 1974, FNUC, IHFP, IH 017.
36 McClintock, *The Old North Trail,* 235-36.
37 Peacock, "Piikani Ethnobotany," 1.
38 Ibid., 22-23.
39 Joan Scott-Brown, "Stoney Ethnobotany: An Indication of Cultural Change amongst Stoney Women of Morley, Alberta" (master's thesis, University of Calgary, 1977), 13.

40 Peacock, "Piikani Ethnobotany."
41 "Notes on Blackfoot Economics," unpublished manuscript, Glenbow Archives (GA), Oscar Lewis Fonds, M8462, p. 5.
42 Elizabeth Vibert, "Real Men Hunt Buffalo: Masculinity, Race, and Class in British Fur Traders' Narratives," in *Gender and History in Canada*, ed. Joy Parr and Mark Rosenfeld (Mississauga, ON: Copp Clark, 1996), 50-53.
43 Ibid., 52.
44 Patricia Albers, "Introduction: New Perspectives on Plains Indian Women," in *The Hidden Half: Studies of Plains Indian Women*, ed. Patricia Albers and Beatrice Medicine (Lanham, MD: University Press of America, 1983), 1-2.
45 Sarah Carter, "Categories and Terrains of Exclusion: Constructing the 'Indian Woman' in the Early Settlement Era in Western Canada," *Great Plains Quarterly* 13 (Summer 1993): 148. See also Adele Perry, *On the Edge of Empire: Gender, Race, and the Making of British Columbia, 1849-1872* (Toronto: University of Toronto Press, 2001).
46 Sarah Carter, "First Nations Women and Colonization on the Canadian Prairies, 1870s-1920s," in *Rethinking Canada: The Promise of Women's History*, edited by Veronica Strong-Boag, Mona Gleason, and Adele Perry, 4th ed. (Don Mills, ON: Oxford University Press, 2002), 135-48.
47 Wissler, *Social Organization and Ritualistic Ceremonies*, 28.
48 Ibid.
49 Ibid.

Chapter 3: Giving Birth

1 Sarah Carter, *Capturing Women: The Manipulation of Cultural Imagery in Canada's Prairie West* (Montreal/Kingston: McGill-Queen's University Press, 1997), 5.
2 Ibid., 9. See also Joan Jensen, *Calling This Place Home: Women on the Wisconsin Frontier, 1850-1925* (Minneapolis: Minnesota Historical Society Press, 2006).
3 Barbara Handy-Marchello, *Women of the Northern Plains: Gender and Settlement on the Homestead Frontier, 1870-1930* (Minneapolis: Minnesota Historical Society Press, 2005), 27-52.
4 Gerald Friesen, *The Canadian Prairies: A History* (Toronto: University of Toronto Press, 1987), 242.
5 Canada, *Census of Canada, 1880-81*, vol. 1 (Ottawa: Maclean, Roger, 1882), 300-1.
6 Howard Palmer and Tamara Palmer, *Alberta: A New History* (Edmonton: Hurtig, 1990), 50-51.
7 Ibid., 68.
8 Canada, *Census of Canada, 1901* (Ottawa: King's Printer, 1903), 392-93.
9 Palmer and Palmer, *Alberta: A New History*, 76-77.
10 Canada, *Census of Canada, 1921* (Ottawa: King's Printer, 1924), 329, 255; Canada, *Census of Canada, 1931* (Ottawa: King's Printer, 1936), 820.
11 Palmer and Palmer, *Alberta: A New History*, 124-25.
12 Canada, *Census of the North-West Provinces, 1906* (Ottawa: King's Printer, 1907), 102.
13 Ibid.
14 Canada, *Census of Canada, 1921*, 197-200.
15 Anne Woywitka, "Pioneers in Sickness and in Health," *Alberta History* 49, 1 (2001): 16.

16 Pioneer Questionnaire, File 8, Health, Saskatchewan Archives Board (SAB), X.2: Mrs. Maggie Whyte, 1883, and Mrs. Ellen W. Hubbard, 1894; Lesley Biggs, "Rethinking the History of Midwifery in Canada," in *Reconceiving Midwifery*, ed. Ivy Bourgeault, Cecilia Benoit, and Robbi Davis-Floyd (Montreal/Kingston: McGill-Queen's University Press, 2004), 17-45; Susan Smith, *Japanese American Midwives: Culture, Community, and Health Politics, 1880-1950* (Urbana: University of Illinois Press, 2005), 101.

17 Susan Smith, "White Nurses, Black Midwives, and Public Health in Mississippi, 1920-1950," *Nursing History Review* 2 (1994): 30-31.

18 Ibid., 31.

19 Wendy Mitchinson, *Giving Birth in Canada, 1900-1950* (Toronto: University of Toronto Press, 2002), 168.

20 Karen Flint, "Competition, Race, and Professionalization: African Healers and White Healers in Natal, South Africa, in the Early Twentieth Century," *Social History of Medicine* 14, 2 (2001): 199-221.

21 Ibid., 209-10.

22 Smith, "White Nurses, Black Midwives," 30-31.

23 W.H. Long, ed., *Fort Pelly Journal of Daily Occurrences, 1863* (Regina: Regina Archaeological Society, 1987), 128. Fort Pelly was at the northeast elbow of the Assiniboine River, eight miles west of the present-day village of Pelly, Saskatchewan. It was built in 1824, burned down in 1842-43, rebuilt, and then moved to another location in 1856-57. The fort was closed in 1912.

24 John Webster Grant, *Moon of Wintertime: Missionaries and the Indians of Canada in Encounter since 1534* (Toronto: University of Toronto Press, 1984), 105.

25 S.A. Archer, ed., *A Heroine of the North: Memoirs of Charlotte Selina Bompas, 1830-1917* (London: Society for Promoting Christian Knowledge, 1929), 74.

26 Ibid., 75-76.

27 Ibid.

28 Myra Rutherdale, "Revisiting Colonization through Gender: Anglican Missionary Women in the Pacific Northwest and the Arctic, 1860-1945," *BC Studies*, no. 104 (Winter 1994): 15. See also Rutherdale, *Women and the White Man's God: Gender and Race in the Canadian Mission Field* (Vancouver: UBC Press, 2002), 43-49.

29 *Moosomin: Century One Town and Country* (Altona, MB: D.W. Friesen, 1981), 4.

30 Ibid.

31 Kate Brighty Colley, *While Rivers Flow: Stories of Early Alberta* (Saskatoon: Western Producer, 1970), 56-57, 61; Irene Stewart, ed., *These Were Our Yesterdays: A History of District Nursing in Alberta* (Calgary: Friesen, 1979), 15-29.

32 François Adam, "Duhamel," *Alberta Folklore Quarterly* 1, 1 (1945): 14-15.

33 Ibid.

34 Nanci Langford, "Childbirth on the Canadian Prairies, 1880-1930," in *Telling Tales: Essays in Western Women's History*, ed. Catherine Cavanaugh and Randi Warne (Vancouver: UBC Press, 2000), 148-49.

35 "The Story of My Life, 1868-1940," unpublished manuscript, SAB, Effie Storer Papers, p. 24.

36 Lester Peterson, *The Story of the Sechelt Nation* (Sechelt, BC: Sechelt Indian Band, 1990), 100-1.

37 Stephen Hume, *Lilies and Fireweed: Frontier Women of British Columbia* (Madeira Park, BC: Harbour Publishing, 2004), 73-76.

38 Margaret Ormsby, ed., *A Pioneer Gentlewoman in British Columbia: The Recollections of Susan Allison* (Vancouver: UBC Press, 1976), 28.
39 Ibid.
40 Ibid., 60.
41 Emmy Preston, ed., *Pioneers of Grandview District* (Steinbach, MB: Carillon, 1976), 103.
42 Ibid., 102-3.
43 Langford, "Childbirth on the Canadian Prairies," 156.
44 Helen MacMurchy, *Maternal Mortality in Canada* (Ottawa: Department of Health, 1928), 23.
45 Jacalyn Duffin, *Langstaff: A Nineteenth-Century Medical Life* (Toronto: University of Toronto Press, 1993).
46 "Treaty Indians and Doctors," Glenbow Archives (GA), George H. Gooderham Family Fonds, M4738, box 2, file 12, p. 2.
47 "The Story of My Life, 1868-1940," p. 10.
48 Ibid., 11.
49 Maureen Lux, Assiniboine field notes, Kay Thompson interview, January 1998, cited in Maureen Lux, *Medicine That Walks: Disease, Medicine, and Canadian Plains Native People, 1880-1940* (Toronto: University of Toronto Press, 2001), 95-96.
50 Frog Lake Community Club, *Land of Red and White* (Heinsburg, AB: 1977), 98.
51 Regina Flannery, *Ellen Smallboy: Glimpses of a Cree Woman's Life* (Montreal/Kingston: McGill-Queen's University Press, 1995), 51.
52 Veronica Strong-Boag and Kathryn McPherson, "The Confinement of Women: Childbirth and Hospitalization in Vancouver, 1919-1930," *BC Studies*, nos. 69 and 70 (Spring-Summer 1986): 147.
53 Ibid.
54 Pioneer Questionnaire, SAB, X.2: Mrs. Priscilla Spencer, 1878; Esther Maud Goldsmith, 1884; and Robert Diguid, 1902.
55 Memorial University of Newfoundland Folklore and Language Archive, no. 79-549, Debbie G.J. Hallett, "Irene (Farwell) Bradley: The Art of Midwifery," 11-12, cited in Mitchinson, *Giving Birth in Canada*, 69.
56 Pioneer Questionnaire, SAB, X.2: Ethel Jameson, 1901; Winnifred Taylor, 1903; Charles Birdsell Riley, 1904; Isabella Hallam, 1905; and Mary Archer, 1907.
57 Ibid., Ethel Jameson, 1901.
58 Ibid., Winnifred Taylor, 1903.
59 Biggs, "Rethinking the History of Midwifery," 29-36.
60 MacMurchy, *Maternal Mortality in Canada*, 12.
61 Pioneer Questionnaire, SAB, X.2: Mrs. Mary E. Bishop, 1880; Herbert Booth, 1883; Charles Bray, 1882; Jane Marmichael, 1887; Ella Mott, 1887; and Isabella Hallam, 1905. Given the expense and inconvenience, doctors were considered the last resort.
62 M.G. McCallum, "The Alberta Department of Public Health," in *The Federal and Provincial Health Services in Canada,* ed. R.D. Defries, 2nd ed. (Ottawa: Canadian Public Health Association, 1962), 110.
63 Pioneer Questionnaire, SAB, X.2: Mrs. Ellen Hubbard, 1894, and Mrs. Maggie Whyte, 1883.
64 Ibid., Mrs. Jane Marmichael, 1887.
65 Regina Women's Canadian Club Convention, 1924, Essays on Pioneer Days, SAB, R-176, II22.

66 Flannery, *Ellen Smallboy*, 32.
67 Laurel Halladay, "We'll See You Next Year: Maternity Homes in Southern Saskatchewan in the First Half of the Twentieth Century" (master's thesis, Carleton University, 1996), 1-3.
68 Pioneer Questionnaire, SAB, X.2: Winnifred Taylor, 1903.
69 Mitchinson, *Giving Birth in Canada*, 173.
70 MacMurchy, *Maternal Mortality in Canada*, 23.
71 Pioneer Questionnaire, SAB, X.2: Edith Mary Stillborne, 1883.
72 Mitchinson, *Giving Birth in Canada*, 173-78.
73 Pioneer Questionnaire, SAB, X.2: Ella Mott, 1887.
74 Lux, *Medicine That Walks*, 98.
75 For an account of the accident, see John Julius Martin, *The Prairie Hub: An Outline of Early Western Events from the Hand Hills to the Buffalo Hills* (Rosebud, AB: Strathmore Standard, 1967), 179. For information regarding Rundle's life and work, see Frits Pannekoek, "Robert T. Rundle," *Dictionary of Canadian Biography Online*.
76 John Maclean, February 29, 1888, United Church of Canada (UCC), Victoria College Archives (VCA), John Maclean Papers, Diaries and Notebooks, box 11, file 5.
77 Ibid.
78 Ibid., file 4, December 13, 1886.
79 Adam, "Duhamel," 14-15. See also UCC, VCA, John Maclean Papers, Diaries and Notebooks, box 11, file 5, February 29, 1888.
80 Marie Rose Smith, "My Eighty Years on the Plains," unpublished manuscript, GA, Marie Rose Smith Fonds, M1154, file 4, pp. 44-45.
81 Martin, *The Prairie Hub*, 179.
82 Pioneer Questionnaire, SAB, X2: Charles Cantlon Bray, 1883, Wolseley, Saskatchewan.
83 Canada, *Census of Canada, 1880-81*, vol. 1 (Ottawa: Maclean, Roger, 1882), 94-95, 300-1.
84 Rod Bantjes, *Improved Earth: Prairie Space as Modern Artefact, 1869-1944* (Toronto: University of Toronto Press, 2005), 58.
85 Elizabeth Bailey Price, "Pioneers of the Foothills," *Maclean's Magazine*, July 1, 1927, 85; Annie McDougall, "Pioneer Life in the 1870s," *Alberta History* 46, 2 (1998): 26.
86 Price, "Pioneers of the Foothills."
87 F.C. Cornish, "Recollections and Papers as a Pioneer Indian Agent," GA, F.C. Cornish Fonds, M266, p. 13.
88 Ibid.
89 Eliane Leslau Silverman, *The Last Best West: Women on the Alberta Frontier, 1880-1930* (Calgary: Fifth House, 1998), 84-85.
90 Sheila McManus, *The Line Which Separates: Race, Gender, and the Making of the Alberta-Montana Borderlands* (Lincoln: University of Nebraska Press, 2005), 149.
91 Monica Hopkins, *Letters from a Lady Rancher* (Halifax: Formac Publishing, 1982), 81-83.
92 Ibid., 79.
93 Canada, *Annual Report of the Department of Indian Affairs (1896)*, 152; Canada, *Annual Report of the Department of Indian Affairs (1897)*, 132, 136, 168; Canada, *Annual Report of the Department of Indian Affairs (1899)*, 129.
94 Canada, *Annual Report of the Department of Indian Affairs (1891)*, 54; Canada, *Annual Report of the Department of Indian Affairs (1897)*, 135, 168; Canada, *Annual Report of the Department of Indian Affairs (1898)*, 125, 128. Agents often noted that Aboriginal men were employed by the NWMP to haul supplies of coal and lumber. Canada, *Annual Report of*

the Department of Indian Affairs for the Year Ending June 30, 1900 (Ottawa: Queen's Printer, 1901), 137, 138, 179; Canada, *Annual Report of the Department of Indian Affairs for the Year Ending June 30, 1905* (Ottawa: Queen's Printer, 1906), 113, 114, 116, 153. The Nakoda worked seasonally in the lumber industry. Pringle, Stoney Agent, to Scott, April 28, 1927, Library and Archives Canada (LAC), RG 29, National Health and Welfare, vol. 3403, box 229, file 823-1-A772. For a detailed account of Aboriginal participation in southern Alberta's economy, see W. Keith Regular, *Neighbours and Networks: The Blood Tribe in the Southern Alberta Economy, 1884-1939* (Calgary: University of Calgary Press, 2009).

95 Canada, *Annual Report* (1891), 54; Canada, *Annual Report* (1897), 135, 168; Canada, *Annual Report* (1898), 125, 128; Canada, *Annual Report* (1900), 137, 138, 179; Canada, *Annual Report* (1905), 113, 114, 116, 153.

96 Simon Evans, *The Bar U: Canadian Ranching History* (Calgary: University of Calgary Press, 2004), 259-63.

97 Address delivered by Mrs. (Rev.) John McDougall at the evening service of the Pincher Creek United Church, June 16, 1935, GA, McDougall Family Fonds, M729, file 21.

98 F.C. Cornish, "Recollections and Papers as a Pioneer Indian Agent," 13.

99 John Maclean, *Canadian Savage Folk: The Native Tribes of Canada* (Toronto: W. Briggs, 1896), 201. Nor did Maclean reveal in his many publications, which catalogued the cultures of North American Aboriginal people, the effectiveness of certain treatments used by Aboriginal healers.

100 For examples of Maclean's writing, see *The Indians of Canada: Their Manners and Customs* (Toronto: William Briggs, 1907); *H.B. Steinhauer: His Work among the Cree Indians of the Western Canadian Plains* (Toronto: William Briggs, n.d.); *McDougall of Alberta* (Toronto: Ryerson, 1927); and *Vanguards of Canada* (Toronto: Missionary Society of the Methodist Church, 1918).

101 Jennifer S.H. Brown, "A Cree Nurse in a Cradle of Methodism: Little Mary and the Egerton R. Young Family at Norway House and Berens River," in *Canadian Family History: Selected Readings*, ed. Bettina Bradbury (Toronto: Copp Clark Pitman, 1992), 90-110. The wife of Methodist missionary Egerton Ryerson Young similarly relied on the help of a Cree woman named Little Mary to care for her children during the family's tenure in the West. Little Mary does not appear in any of Young's writings. It was not until shortly before his death that Eddie, one of the children Little Mary cared for, wrote about his affection for her.

102 Andrea Smith, *Conquest: Sexual Violence and American Indian Genocide* (Cambridge: South End, 2005), 9.

103 Katherine Pettipas, *Severing the Ties That Bind: Government Repression of Indigenous Religious Ceremonies on the Prairies* (Winnipeg: University of Manitoba Press, 1994), 87-125.

104 Ibid., 88.

105 For examples of literature on colonialism that looks at Aboriginal women and domesticity, see V.L. Rafael, *Colonial Domesticity: White Women and US Rule in the Philippines* (Durham, NC: Duke University Press, 1995). V.L. Rafael, "Colonial Domesticity: Engendering Race at the Edge of Empire, 1899-1920," in *White Love and Other Events in Filipino History*, ed. V.L. Rafael (Durham, NC: Duke University Press, 2007), 52-75. Jean Comaroff and John Comaroff, "Homemade Hegemony: Modernity, Domesticity, and Colonialism in South Africa," in *African Encounters with Domesticity*, ed. Karen Tranberg Hansen (New Jersey: Rutgers, 1992), 37-74; Antoinette Burton, *Burdens of History: British Feminists, Indian Women, and Imperial Culture, 1865-1915* (London: University of North Carolina Press, 1994); and Margaret Jacobs, "Working on the Domestic Frontier: American Indian Domestic

Servants in White Women's Household in the San Francisco Area, 1920-1940," *Frontiers* 28, 1-2 (2007): 165-99.
106 L. Vankoughnet to Macdonald, November 15, 1883, LAC, RG 10, Department of Indian Affairs, vol. 1009, file 628, pp. 596-635; see also Carter, *Capturing Women*, 187-88.
107 Sarah Carter, "Categories and Terrains of Exclusion: Constructing the 'Indian Woman' in the Early Settlement Era in Western Canada," in *Telling Tales: Essays in Western Women's History*, ed. Catherine Cavanaugh and Randi Warne (Vancouver: UBC Press, 2000), 76-77.
108 Constance Backhouse, "Nineteenth-Century Canadian Prostitution Law: Reflection of a Discriminatory Society," *Social History/Histoire sociale* 18, 36 (1985): 422; Carter, *Capturing Women*, 169-81.
109 Carter, "Categories and Terrains of Exclusion," 77.
110 Nanci Langford, "Childbirth on the Canadian Prairies," 147-73.

Chapter 4: Converging Therapeutic Systems

1 Meagan Vaughan, *Curing Their Ills: Colonial Power and African Illness* (Palo Alto, CA: Stanford University Press, 1991), 56-57.
2 John Webster Grant, *Moon of Wintertime: Missionaries and Indians of Canada in Encounter since 1534* (Toronto: University of Toronto Press, 1984), 145.
3 Ibid., 162.
4 C.L. Higham, "'A Hewer of Wood and Drover of Water': Expectations of Protestant Missionary Women on the Western Frontiers of Canada and the United States, 1830-1900," *Canadian Review of American Studies* 31, 1 (2001): 447.
5 Rosemary Gagan, "Gender, Work, and Zeal: Women Missionaries in Canada and Abroad," *Labour/Le Travail* 53 (2004): 1.
6 Christin Hancock, "Sovereign Bodies: Women, Health Care, and Federal Indian Policy, 1890-1986" (PhD diss., Brown University, 2006), 50.
7 Grant, *Moon of Wintertime*, 155.
8 Treaty 7 Elders and Tribal Council et al., *The True Spirit and Original Intent of Treaty 7* (Montreal/Kingston: McGill-Queen's University Press, 1996), 52.
9 John Maclean to Annie Maclean, March 18, 1889, United Church of Canada (UCC), Victoria College Archives (VCA), John Maclean Papers, Correspondence, box 1, file 7.
10 Grant, *Moon of Wintertime*, 146. See also Pauline Paul, "A History of the Edmonton General Hospital, 1895-1970: 'Be Faithful to the Duties of Your Calling'" (PhD diss., University of Alberta, 1994), 29.
11 Robert Choquette, *The Oblate Assault on Canada's Northwest* (Ottawa: University of Ottawa Press, 1995), 93.
12 Myra Rutherdale, *Women and the White Man's God: Gender and Race in the Canadian Mission Field* (Vancouver: UBC Press, 2003), 19.
13 Blackfoot Agent Pocklington to Inspector of Agencies, June 8, 1895; P. Baker to Inspector of Agencies, June 6, 1895; Lucius Hardyman to Inspector of Agencies, n.d.; Blackfoot Agent Begg to DIA, May 2, 1895; Tims to DIA, May 3, 1895; Blackfoot Agent Begg to DIA, May 2, 1895, Library and Archives Canada (LAC), RG 10, Department of Indian Affairs, vol. 3928, file 117,004-1.
14 H.W. Gibbon Stocken, *Among the Blackfoot and Sarcee*, edited by Hugh Dempsey (Calgary: Glenbow Museum, 1976), 21.

15 "Old Anglican Boarding School Now Sanatorium," *Calgary Herald,* November 17, 1921.
16 John Maclean, "Among the Indians," n.d, UCC, VCA, John Maclean Papers, Minor Publications, box 33, file 267.
17 Kate Brown, "Peigan Reserve, Fort Macleod," *Letter Leaflet,* March 1891, 198, and December 1888, 5, General Synod Archives (GSA), Anglican Church of Canada (ACC), Missionary Society Papers (MSP).
18 Kate Brown, "Gleichen," *Letter Leaflet,* January 1889, 5, and Miss Garlick, *Letter Leaflet,* October 1899, 412-13.
19 Mrs. Bourne, "Peigan Reserve," *Letter Leaflet,* February 1890, 6-7; "Letter to Mrs. Grindlay," *Letter Leaflet,* September 1890, 124-25; and "Peigan Indian House, Fort Macleod," *Letter Leaflet,* January 1892, 18-20.
20 H.W. Gibbon Stocken, "Report of St. John's Hospital, Blackfoot Reserve," *Letter Leaflet,* December 1896, 47. Opthalmia is a painful and periodic swelling of the conjunctiva, which is the mucous membrane that lines the inner surface of the eyelids and continues over the forepart of the eyeball.
21 Mrs. Bourne, "Letters from Missionaries," *Letter Leaflet,* September 1890, 12.
22 Kate Brown, "Letters from Missionaries," *Letter Leaflet,* June 1896, 654.
23 Miss Essam, *Letter Leaflet,* July 1898, 298.
24 Canada, *Annual Report of the Department of Indian Affairs (1899),* 129; Canada, *Annual Report of the Department of Indian Affairs (1898),* 159; Sarah Carter, "First Nations Women and Colonization on the Canadian Prairies, 1870s-1920s," in *Rethinking Canada: The Promise of Women's History,* ed. Veronica Strong-Boag, Mona Gleason, and Adele Perry, 4th ed. (Don Mills, ON: Oxford University Press, 2002), 141. See also John Lutz, "Gender and Work in Lekwammen Families, 1843-1970," in *Gendered Pasts: Historical Essays in Femininity and Masculinity in Canada,* ed. Kathryn McPherson, Cecilia Morgan, and Nancy Forestell (Don Mills, ON: Oxford University Press, 1999), 94.
25 Blood letter books, January 14, 1895, LAC, RG 10, vol. 1560.
26 Mr. Stocken, "News from the Field," *Letter Leaflet,* May 1904, 260.
27 Kate Brown, "Blackfoot Reserve, Gleichen," *Letter Leaflet,* November 1888, 6, and "Gleichen," *Letter Leaflet,* November 1889, 5-6.
28 "Letters from Missionaries," *Letter Leaflet,* January 1889, 4.
29 "Gleichen," *Letter Leaflet,* November 1888, 7-8.
30 "Peigan Reserve," *Letter Leaflet,* March 1891, 64.
31 "Letter from the Blackfoot Hospital," *Letter Leaflet,* May 1904, 260.
32 Ibid.
33 Canada, *Annual Report (1899),* 129; Canada, *Annual Report (1898),* 159. Carter, "First Nations Women and Colonization," 141; Elizabeth Churchill, "Tsuu T'ina: A History of a First Nations Community" (PhD diss., University of Calgary, 1994), 101.
34 Lutz, "Gender and Work in Lekwammen Families," 94.
35 Ibid.
36 Carter, "First Nations Women and Colonization," 141.
37 Ibid., 142; see also Annora Brown, *Old Man's Garden* (Toronto: Dent, 1954).
38 Mrs. J.A. Reid, "The Neighbourhood of Battleford," Saskatchewan Archives Board, Regina Women's Canadian Club Conventions, 1924: Essays on Pioneer Days, R-176 II, no. 15.
39 Ibid.
40 Published letters regarding mission work among Blood – newspaper unknown, UCC, VCA, John Maclean Papers, minor publications, box 33, file 267.

41 Notes on Mrs. Eliza Boyd McDougall, City of Edmonton Archives (CEA), MS10, Edna Kells Manuscripts, box 2, file 64, p. 8.
42 Miss Buehler, "Our New Work and Worker among the Indians," *Missionary Outlook*, October 1904, 240.
43 Adele Perry, "From 'the Hot-Bed of Vice' to the 'Good and Well-Ordered Christian Home': First Nations' Housing and Reform in Nineteenth-Century British Columbia," *Ethnohistory* 50, 4 (2003): 588.
44 Margaret Laing, "Morley Hospital," *Christian Guardian*, August 7, 1907, 16.
45 Brian Titley, *The Indian Commissioners: Agents of the State and Indian Policy in Canada's Prairie West, 1873-1932* (Edmonton: University of Alberta Press, 2009), 93-120.
46 Report, Hayter Reed, March 14, 1892, LAC, RG 10, vol. 3870, file 88706.
47 Miss Barker, "McDougall Orphanage," *Missionary Outlook*, August 1885, 124.
48 Kate Brown, "Letters from Missionaries," *Letter Leaflet*, June 1895, 654. Scrofula is a form of tuberculosis that affects the lymph glands in the neck. It can result in the appearance of painful lesions.
49 Untitled article, author not given, *Letter Leaflet*, February 1890, 6.
50 Mary-Ellen Kelm, *Colonizing Bodies: Aboriginal Health and Healing in British Columbia, 1900-1950* (Vancouver: UBC Press, 1998), 153.
51 Report on Indian Missions," 1900, p. 6, University of Calgary, Special Collections (UCSC), Anglican Church of Canada, Calgary Diocese.
52 Secretary of the CMS to Rev. Tims, February 19, 1897, Glenbow Archives (GA), Anglican Church, Calgary Indian Missions, Incoming Correspondence, M1356, file 2.
53 Rev. Tims to Mr. O'Meara of the CMS, March 1, 1897, ibid.
54 Judith Young, "'Monthly' Nurses, Sick Nurses, and Midwives in 19th-Century Toronto," *Canadian Bulletin of Medical History/Bulletin canadien d'histoire* 21, 2 (2004): 296-97.
55 Pauline Paul, "A History of the Edmonton General Hospital: 1895-1970" (PhD diss., University of Alberta, 1994), 35.
56 Janet Ross-Kerr, *Prepared to Care: Nurses and Nursing in Alberta* (Edmonton: University of Alberta Press, 1998), 20.
57 Tony Cashman, *Heritage of Service: The History of Nursing in Alberta* (Edmonton: Alberta Association of Registered Nurses, 1966), 21.
58 Ibid.
59 Paul, "A History of the Edmonton General Hospital," 21, 35.
60 Cashman, *Heritage of Service*, 23-36.
61 Ross-Kerr, *Prepared to Care*, 21.
62 Cashman, *Heritage of Service*, 21, 35.
63 Sarah Carter, *Aboriginal People and Colonizers of Western Canada to 1900* (Toronto: University of Toronto Press, 1999), 112.
64 Hugh Shewell, *Enough to Keep Them Alive: Indian Social Welfare in Canada, 1873-1965* (Toronto: University of Toronto Press, 2004), 30-31.
65 Hayter Reed to Sarcee Agent Cornish, March 12, 1877, LAC, RG 10, series A, vol. 1630.
66 Deputy Superintendent of Indian Affairs to Macdonald, September 30, 1885, LAC, RG 10, vol. 3632, file 6326; Incoming Correspondence, Hayter Reed to Sarcee Agent Cornish, March 12, 1887, and March 24, 1887, LAC, RG 10, vol. 1630.
67 J.D. McLean to Sarcee Agent McNeill, January 24, 1899, LAC, RG 10, vol. 1627; Incoming Correspondence, Assistant Indian Commissioner to Sarcee Agent Cornish, February 4, 1890, LAC, RG 10, vol. 1624; Incoming Correspondence, Indian Commissioner to Sarcee Agent Lucas, February 27, 1893, LAC, RG 10, vol. 1626.

68 Agent Lucas, March 3, 1893, LAC, RG 10, vol. 1641.
69 Alexander Morris, *The Treaties of Canada with the Indians* (Toronto: Prospero, 2000 [1880]), 177-78; Kathryn McPherson, "Nursing and Colonization: The Work of Indian Health Service Nurses in Manitoba," in *Women, Health, and Nation: Canada and the United States since 1945*, ed. Georgina Feldberg et al. (Montreal/Kingston: McGill-Queen's University Press, 2003), 226-27.
70 Deputy Superintendent General of Indian Affairs to Sir John A. Macdonald, September 30, 1885, LAC, RG 10, vol. 3632, file 6326; Incoming Correspondence, Hayter Reed to Sarcee Agent Cornish, March 12, 1877, LAC, RG 10, vol. 1630.
71 R.B. Nevitt, *A Winter at Fort Macleod*, edited by Hugh Dempsey (Calgary: Glenbow-Alberta Institute, 1974), 70.
72 Petition, Sir John A. Macdonald, May 8, 1883, LAC, RG 10, vol. 3632, file 6326.
73 Edgar Dewdney to Supt. General of Indian Affairs, April 11, 1983, ibid.; Report, Mr. Wadsworth to the Indian Commissioner, May 16, 1881, LAC, RG 10, vol. 3720, file 23-341.
74 Petition, Sir John A. Macdonald, April 1882, LAC, RG 10, vol. 3599, file 1500; Sir John A. Macdonald, April 11 and May 8, 1883, LAC, RG 10, vol. 3632, file 6326.
75 Ibid.
76 Deputy Superintendent of Indian Affairs to Macdonald, September 30, 1885; Edgar Dewdney to Superintendent General of Indian Affairs, November 19, 1885; and Theo White to Sir Hector Langevin, April 11, 1888, LAC, RG 10, vol. 3632, file 6326.
77 White to Langevin, April 11, 1888.
78 Maureen Lux, *Medicine That Walks: Disease, Medicine, and Canadian Plains Native People, 1880-1940* (Toronto: University of Toronto Press, 2001), 143-44.
79 Ibid., 144.
80 White to Langevin, April 11, 1888; Report, Mr. Wadsworth, July 20, 1900, and Blood Agent Wilson to Indian Commissioner, February 2, 1897, LAC, RG 10, vol. 3632, file 6326. See also Lux, *Medicine That Walks*, 143-47.
81 White to Langevin, April 11, 1888.
82 Hayter Reed to Sarcee Agent de Balinhard, March 24, 1887, LAC, RG 10, vol. 1630; Incoming Correspondence, Hayter Reed to Sarcee Agent Cornish, November 19, 1889, LAC, RG 10, vol. 1624.
83 Mary-Ellen Kelm, "Diagnosing the Discursive Indian: Medicine, Gender, and the Dying Race," *Ethnohistory* 52, 2 (2005): 371-406.
84 Sarah Carter, *Lost Harvests: Prairie Indian Reserve Farmers and Government Policy* (Montreal/Kingston: McGill-Queen's University Press, 1990), 15-16.
85 E. Brian Titley, *A Narrow Vision: Duncan Campbell Scott and the Administration of Indian Affairs in Canada* (Vancouver: UBC Press, 1986), 24.
86 Report, Blood Agent Pocklington, June 4, 1890, LAC, RG 10, vol. 3759, file 31949. Comparable evidence can be found in DIA records throughout the 1920s. See, for example, Dr. J.H. Rivers to J. Wilson, Blood Agent Wilson, November 14, 1903, GA, Blood Indian Agency Fonds (DIA), M1788, file 22; McLean to Blood Agent Dilworth, August 12, 1914, LAC, RG 10, vol. 1542; Circular, J.D. McLean to All Medical Officers, December 2, 1919; Blackfoot Agent J.H. Gooderham to High River General Hospital; and Reverend Gibbon Stocken to Blackfoot Indian Agent J.H. Gooderham, February 29, 1912, LAC, RG 10, vol. 1153.
87 J.D. McLean to Sarcee Agent McNeill, January 24, 1899, LAC, RG 10, vol. 1627; Incoming Correspondence, Assistant Indian Commissioner to Sarcee Agent Cornish, February 4, 1890, LAC, RG 10, vol. 1624; Incoming Correspondence, Indian Commissioner to Sarcee Agent Lucas, February 27, 1893, LAC, RG 10, vol. 1626. Similar concerns were even

expressed during the 1918 flu pandemic. See Peigan Agent Gunn to Scott, November 18, 1918, LAC, RG 29, National Health and Welfare, vol. 2919, file 841-1A772, part 1.
88 Cynthia Comacchio, *"Nations Are Built of Babies": Saving Ontario's Mothers and Children, 1900-1940* (Montreal/Kingston: McGill-Queen's University Press, 1993), 92-115; Mariana Valverde, *The Age of Light, Soap, and Water: Moral Reform in English Canada, 1885-1925* (Toronto: McClelland and Stewart, 1991), 129-54.

Chapter 5: Laying the Foundation

1 Nancy Reifel, "American Indian Views of Public Health Nursing, 1930-1950," *American Indian Culture and Research Journal* 23, 3 (1999): 143-54. In a similar cultural context, historian Nancy Reifel found that the Sioux assessed the work of field nurses based on the effectiveness of their medicines and the quality of their character.
2 Gibbon Stocken, *Among the Blackfoot and the Sarcee,* edited by Hugh Dempsey (Calgary: Glenbow Museum, 1987), xiii; the Reverend Gibbon Stocken, *Letter Leaflet,* August 1893, 295.
3 The Reverend Gibbon Stocken, *Letter Leaflet,* August 1893, 295. See also "Blackfoot Hospital Report," *Letter Leaflet,* December 1896, 47.
4 W.R. Haynes, *Letter Leaflet,* September 1899, 373.
5 Miss Garlick, *Letter Leaflet,* October 1899, 412-13.
6 Hayter Reed to the Assistant Indian Commissioner, September 6, 1894, Library and Archives Canada (LAC), RG 10, vol. 3934, file 118-065; Memorandum, A.S. Williams, Acting Deputy Superintendent General of Indian Affairs, to Dr. Harold McGill, December 6, 1935, Glenbow Archives (GA), Harold Wigmore and Emma Griffis McGill Fonds, M742, file 36.
7 Grey Nuns, Personnel et Oeuvre, December 1893 and December 1894, Grey Nuns Archives, Montreal (GNAM), Hopital Notre-Dame-des-Sept-Douleurs/Stand Off, Blood Reserve, Alberta, L049 (hereafter HNDSD), E1; Mr. Wadsworth's Report of the Blood Hospital, August 9, 1894, LAC, RG 10, vol. 3934, file 118-065. The nursing sisters possessed a great deal of experience but no formal training as nurses.
8 Suzanne Olivier, "Historique," 2, GNAM, HNDSD.
9 Report from Canon Stocken, June 1899, University of Calgary, Special Collecions (UCSC), Anglican Church of Canada (ACC), Calgary Diocese (CD), General Files, J.W. Tims, Blackfoot and Sarcee Mission Correspondence, box 8, file 18; Laurie Meijer Drees, "Reserve Hospitals and Medical Officers: Health Care and Indian Peoples in Southern Alberta, 1890s-1930," *Prairie Forum* 21, 2 (1996): 164.
10 Report from Canon Stocken, June 1899.
11 Calgary Indian Missions Report, 1898 to 1901, *Letter Leaflet,* December 1901, 40-41.
12 Drees, "Reserve Hospitals and Medical Officers," 165.
13 Peigan Correspondence, J.D. McLean to Peigan Agent Gunn, April 8, 1915, LAC, RG 10, vol. 1416.
14 Medical Inspection Reports, Dr. O.I. Grain, Peigan Reserve, January 26, 1914, LAC, RG 10, vol. 4077, file 454-016. Maureen Lux, *Medicine That Walks: Disease, Medicine, and Canadian Plains Native People, 1880-1940* (Toronto: University of Toronto Press, 2002), 103.
15 Peigan Correspondence, J.D. McLean to Peigan Agent Gunn, July 13, 1914, and October 16, 1914; Dr. Gillespie to Peigan Agent Gunn, October 21, 1914, LAC, RG 10, vol. 1416.
16 Peigan Correspondence, Peigan Agent Thomas Graham to Miss M.G. Kelly and Miss Marion Kelly, February 1, 1919, LAC, RG 10, vol. 1424.

17 Mr. E. Hockely, "St. Paul's Mission, Blood Reserve," *Letter Leaflet,* December 1896; GSA, Calgary Diocese, Report on Indian Missions, 1898, 10; Mrs. Hardyman, "Bull Horn School, Blood Reserve," *Letter Leaflet,* November 1899.
18 Report on Indian Missions, 1905, GSA, ACC, MSP.
19 Reverend H.W. Gibbon Stocken, "Sarcee Reserve," *Letter Leaflet,* January 1892, 7-8; "St. Barnabas Mission, Sarcee Reserve," *Letter Leaflet,* September 1894, 403; and *Letter Leaflet,* August 1893, 295. Anonymous, "Statement as to the School Work in Connection with the Indian Missions," November 10, 1898, UCSC, ACC, MSP.
20 Secretary of the Canadian Church Missionary Association to Reverend Tims, February 19, 1897, GA, Anglican Church, Calgary Indian Missions, Medical Reports, M1356, file 2; J.D. McLean to Rev. Timms School, April 21, 1915, M1356, file 6; and Sarcee Agent Fleetham to Reverend Tims, April 16, 1915, M1356, file 6. J.D. McLean to Dr. Follett, April 23, 1915, LAC, RG 29, National Health and Welfare, vol. 3403, box 229, file 823-1-A772.
21 Biographical Outline, Miss K. Margaret Laing, United Church of Canada (UCC), Victoria College Archives (VCA); T.E.E. Shore to Miss Laing, 1910, UCC, VCA, Methodist Church Missionary Society, Foreign Department, T.E.E. Shore Papers, fonds 14, box 5, file 103.
22 Miss K. Margaret Laing, "Stoney Reserve, Morley Alberta," *Missionary Outlook,* July 1908.
23 Biographical Outline, Miss K. Margaret Laing; T.E.E. Shore to Miss Laing, 1910, UCC, VCA, T.E.E. Shore Papers, fonds 14, box 5, file 103,.
24 Blood Agent Dilworth to Scott, February 14, 1917, and Dilworth to Dr. Tupper, September 1916, LAC, RG 10, vol. 1541; Dilworth to Scott, April 14, 1916, LAC, RG 10, vol. 1540; Peigan Agent Graham to Graham, May 22, 1922, LAC, RG 10, vol. 1425; Canada, *Annual Report of the Department of Indian Affairs for the Year Ended March 31, 1926* (Ottawa: Queen's Printer, 1927), 10.
25 Peigan Agent Wilson to DIA, February 3, 1901, LAC, RG 10, vol. 3632, file 6326; Peigan Agent Arthur to DIA, April 9, 1923, LAC, RG 10, vol. 1425; Canada, *Annual Report of the Department of Indian Affairs for the Year Ended June 30, 1896* (Ottawa: Queen's Printer, 1897), 202; Canada, *Annual Report of the Department of Indian Affairs for the Year Ended March 31, 1915* (Ottawa: Queen's Printer, 1916), 70; Canada, *Annual Report of the Department of Indian Affairs for the Year Ended March 31, 1926* (Ottawa: Queen's Printer, 1927), 10.
26 Brian Titley, *A Narrow Vision: Duncan Campbell Scott and the Administration of Indian Affairs in Canada* (Vancouver: UBC Press, 1986), 83.
27 Megan Sproule-Jones, "Crusading for the Forgotten: Dr. Peter Bryce, Public Health, and Prairie Residential Schools," *Canadian Bulletin of Medical History/Bulletin canadien d'histoire de la médecine* 12, 2 (1996): 205.
28 P.H. Bryce, *Report on the Indian Schools of Manitoba and the Northwest Territories* (Ottawa: Government Printing Bureau, 1907).
29 Sproule-Jones, "Crusading for the Forgotten," 210.
30 Titley, *A Narrow Vision,* 82.
31 Lux, *Medicine That Walks,* 138-39.
32 Canadian Tuberculosis Association, Annual Reports, 1906, 26-27, LAC, Records of the Canadian Tuberculosis Association, vol. 23; Bryce, *Report,* 18. For accounts of conditions in residential schools that contributed to the spread of tuberculosis, see John Milloy, *A National Crime: The Canadian Government and the Residential School System, 1879 to 1986* (Winnipeg: University of Manitoba Press, 1999), 77-107; see also Mary-Ellen Kelm, "A Scandalous Procession: Residential Schooling and the Re/formation of Aboriginal Bodies, 1900-1950," *Native Studies Review* 11, 2 (1996): 62-63.

33 Sproule-Jones, "Crusading for the Forgotten," 211.
34 Florence Melchior, "Nursing Student Labour, Education, and Patient Care at the Medicine Hat General Hospital, Alberta, 1890-1930" (PhD diss., University of Calgary, 2004), 131-36.
35 Kathryn McPherson, *Bedside Matters: The Transformation of Canadian Nursing, 1900-1990* (Toronto: Oxford University Press, 1996), 27.
36 Tony Cashman, *Heritage of Service: The History of Nursing in Alberta* (Edmonton: Alberta Association of Registered Nurses, 1966), 25.
37 Pauline Paul, "A History of the Edmonton General Hospital: 1895-1970" (PhD diss., University of Alberta, 1994,) 84.
38 McPherson, *Bedside Matters,* 27.
39 Pauline Paul, "The Contribution of the Grey Nuns to the Development of Nursing in Canada: Historiographical Issues," *Canadian Bulletin of Medical History/Bulletin canadien d'histoire de la médecine* 11 (1994): 208; McPherson, *Bedside Matters,* 28.
40 Paul, "The Contribution of the Grey Nuns," 209.
41 Emily Cummings to Hayter Reed, January 21, 1897, LAC, RG 10, vol. 3909, file 107-557.
42 Gibbon Stocken to Blackfoot Agent J.H. Gooderham, December 8, 1913, ibid.
43 Rosemary Gagan, *A Sensitive Independence: Canadian Methodist Women Missionaries in Canada and the Orient, 1881-1925* (Montreal/Kingston: McGill-Queen's University Press, 1992); Ruth Brouwer, *New Women for God: Canadian Presbyterian Women and India Missions, 1876-1914* (Toronto: University of Toronto Press, 1990).
44 James Waldram, D. Ann Herring, and T. Kue Young, *Aboriginal Health in Canada: Historical, Cultural, and Epidemiological Perspectives,* 2nd ed. (Toronto: University of Toronto Press, 2006).
45 Laurie Meijer Drees and Lesley McBain, "Nursing and Native Peoples in Northern Saskatchewan, 1930-1950s," *Canadian Bulletin of Medical History/Bulletin canadien d'histoire de la médecine* 18 (2001): 43-65; Kathryn McPherson, "Nursing and Colonization: The Work of Indian Health Services in Manitoba," in *Women, Health, and Nation: Canada and the United States since 1945,* ed. Georgina Feldberg et al. (Montreal/Kingston: McGill-Queen's University Press, 2003), 223-46.
46 Drees and McBain, "Nursing and Native Peoples," 62; McPherson, "Nursing and Colonization," 240-41.
47 Kristin Burnett, "Aboriginal and White Women in the Publications of John Maclean, Egerton Ryerson Young, and John McDougall," in *Unsettled Pasts: Reconceiving the West through Women's History,* ed. Sarah Carter et al. (Calgary: University of Calgary Press, 2005), 103-4.
48 Myra Rutherdale, *Women and the White Man's God: Gender and Race in the Canadian Mission Field* (Vancouver: UBC Press, 2002), 4-5.
49 Gagan, *A Sensitive Independence;* Brouwer, *New Women for God;* Marta Danylewycz, *Taking the Veil: An Alternative to Marriage, Motherhood, and Spinsterhood in Quebec, 1840-1920* (Toronto: McClelland and Stewart, 1987); Elizabeth Gillian Muir and Marilyn Fardig Whiteley, "Introduction: Putting Together the Puzzle of Canadian Women's Christian Work," in *Changing Roles of Women within the Christian Church in Canada,* ed. Elizabeth Gillian Muir and Marilyn Fardig Whiteley (Toronto: University of Toronto Press, 1995), 3-16; Rutherdale, *Women and the White Man's God.*
50 Field matrons, the female equivalent of male farm instructors, were hired to provide Aboriginal women with instruction about European concepts of domesticity and child care.

For a detailed discussion of the Field Matron program, see Lisa Emmerich, "To Respect and Love and Seek the Ways of White Women: Field Matrons, the Office of Indian Affairs, and Civilization Policy, 1890-1938" (PhD diss., University of Maryland, 1987), 25.
51 Alma Booth to Toronto Women's Auxiliary, August 1899, GA, Alice Turner Fonds, M2463; Isabel Turner to Mrs. Cummings, Toronto Women's Auxiliary, June 23, 1897, LAC, RG 10, vol. 3909, file 107-557.
52 Mariana Valverde, *The Age of Light, Soap, and Water: Moral Reform in English Canada, 1885-1925* (Toronto: McClelland and Stewart, 1991), 46-47.
53 Myra Rutherdale, "She Was a Ragged Little Thing: Missionaries, Embodiment, and Refashioning Aboriginal Womanhood in Northern Canada," in *Contact Zones: Aboriginal and Settler Women in Canada's Colonial Past,* ed. Katie Pickles and Myra Rutherdale (Vancouver: UBC Press, 2005), 231.
54 Isabel Turner to Mrs. Cummings, Toronto Women's Auxiliary, June 23, 1897, LAC, RG 10, vol. 3909, file 107-557.
55 G. Smith, Inspector of Construction, to Blood Agent J.E. Ostrauder, May 17, 1924, LAC, RG 10, vol. 1542.
56 Sr. Superior to Father Guy, February 17, 1927, LAC, RG 29, National Health and Welfare.
57 Reverend General to Sister Superior, June 20, 1928, GNAM, HNDSD, Doc. 180.
58 Blood Agent Dilworth to Scott, April 14, 1916, LAC, RG 10, vol. 1540.
59 Fanny Esam to Toronto Women's Auxiliary, August 21, 1899, GA, M2463.
60 Isabel Turner to Mrs. Cummings, Toronto Women's Auxiliary, June 23, 1897; *Letter Leaflet,* February 1899, 127.
61 Jane Megarry, diary, n.d., GA, Jane Megarry Fonds, M4096, file 2.
62 Miss Murray, "News from the Field," *Letter Leaflet,* October 1911, 363.
63 Alma Booth, August 21, 1899, GA, M2463; Report from Blackfoot Agent George Gooderham regarding the Blackfoot Hospital, February 18, 1926, LAC, RG 29, vol. 2592, file 800-1-0443.
64 Mrs. Stanley Stocken, "News from the Field," *Letter Leaflet,* October 1903, 437, GSA, ACC, MSP; Blackfoot Correspondence, Paget, N.W. Commissioner of Indian Affairs to the Blackfoot Agent Wheatley, May 3, 1897, LAC, RG 10, vol. 1154.
65 Milloy, *A National Crime,* 77-128.
66 Marchmont Ing, "Reminiscence," p. 42, UCC, VCA, Marchmont Ing Papers, Personal Papers file, box 8.
67 *Letter Leaflet,* October 1899, 403, and Miss Esam, *Letter Leaflet,* December 1899, 43, GSA, ACC, MSP.
68 Alice Turner, August 21, 1899, GA, M2463.
69 Pamela Margaret White, "Restructuring the Domestic Sphere: Prairie Indian Women on Reserves – Image, Ideology, and State Policy, 1880-1930" (PhD diss., McGill University, 1987), 131-43.
70 Blackfoot Hospital, 1899, GA, Anglican Mission Workers, Letters, M243.
71 Anne McClintock, *Imperial Leather: Race, Gender, and Sexuality in the Colonial Contest* (New York: Routledge, 1995), 170-71.
72 Cynthia Comacchio, *"Nations Are Built of Babies": Saving Ontario's Mothers and Children, 1900-1940* (Montreal/Kingston: McGill-Queen's University Press, 1993), 4. The term *scientific motherhood* refers to social reformers' and the medical profession's attempt, under the guise of nationhood, to use modern child rearing methods to modernize Canadian families in response to the ills of industrialization and urbanization.

73 Canada, *Annual Report (1896)*, 202.
74 Julia Grant, *Raising Baby by the Book: The Education of American Mothers* (London, UK: Yale University Press, 1998), 4.
75 G. Graham-Cumming, "The Health of the Original Canadians, 1867-1967," *Medical Services Journal* 23, 2 (1967): 134.
76 Report on Indian Missions, 1898, p. 12, and 1899, p. 10, UCSC, ACC, CD. Miss Collins, *Letter Leaflet,* October 1899, 403, and *Letter Leaflet,* August 1899, 327.
77 Kate Brown, *Letter Leaflet,* November 1888, 7, and Miss Essam, *Letter Leaflet,* July 1898, 298, GSA.
78 Blood Agency, Dr. Steele to DIA, April 5, 1918, LAC, RG 10, vol. 1541.
79 Blood Hospital, Monthly Medical Reports, June 1911, LAC, RG 10, vol. 1540.
80 Report on Indian Missions, 1897-98, p. 8, and 1899, p. 10; Annual Report of the Women's Auxiliary, Diocese of Toronto, 1911, p. 39, UCSC, ACC, CD.
81 Alice Turner, *Letter Leaflet,* June 1897, 260.
82 Lux, *Medicine That Walks,* 166.
83 School and Hospital Report, February 1913, LAC, RG 10, vol. 1425; Nurse Agnes Huncomb, December 31, 1916, and Nurse Maude Hill, May 1917, GA, Anglican Church, Calgary Indian Missions, Medical Reports, M1356, file 6; Peigan Agent Gunn to W.M. Graham, October 31, 1918, LAC, RG 10, vol. 1424.
84 "Treaty Indians and Doctors," GA, George H. Gooderham Family Fonds, M4738, box 2, file 12, p. 2.
85 Biographical Files, Miss K. Margaret Laing, UCC, VCA.
86 "Reminiscences," Marchmont Ing Papers, box 8, personal papers file, p. 44, UCC, VCA; Miss K. Margaret Laing, "Stoney Reserve, Morley Alberta," *Missionary Outlook,* July 1908.
87 Reifel, "American Indian Views of Public Health," 152. In a similar context, Reifel also found that the Sioux in their interactions with field nurses "took an active role in evaluating and selecting from alternative treatment regimes."
88 Miss K. Margaret Laing, "Morley Hospital," *Missionary Outlook,* August 1907; "Stoney Reserve, Morley Alberta," *Missionary Outlook,* July 1908.
89 Ibid.
90 Supplemental Report Regarding St. Joseph's Industrial School, November 18, 1911, LAC, RG 10, vol. 3933, file 117, pp. 657-61.
91 Ibid.
92 Ibid.; J.D. McLean to Dr. Alfred Ernest Ardiel, February 20, 1913, LAC, RG 10, vol. 3933.
93 Canada, *Annual Reports for the Department of Indian Affairs for the Years Ended June 30, 1881 to March 31, 1906 to March 31, 1918* (Ottawa: Queen's Printer, 1881-1919).
94 Lux, *Medicine that Walks;* Mary-Ellen Kelm, *Colonizing Bodies: Aboriginal Health and Healing in British Columbia, 1900-1950* (Vancouver: UBC Press, 1998).
95 Dr. Lafferty to Clifford Sifton, n.d, LAC, RG 10, vol. 3909, file 107-557.
96 Dr. Lafferty to Clifford Sifton, January 1901, ibid.
97 Memo Superintendent of Indian Affairs James A. Smart, December 29, 1899; Gibbon Stocken to Deputy Superintendent General of Indian Affairs James A. Smart, January 29, 1901; Dr. Lafferty to Minister of the Interior, n.d, ibid.
98 Bishop of St. Albert to Reverend General, January 12, 1913, GNAM, HNDSD, Doc. 125.
99 Blood Agent Julius Hyde to Bishop of St. Albert, January 31, 1913, LAC, RG 10, vol. 1540.

100 Father Renaud to DIA, December 3, 1951, LAC, RG 29, vol. 2609, file 800-1-X444, pt. 1; Megarry, diaries, n.d.; UCSC, Anglican Church, Calgary Diocese Report on Indian Missions, 1899, 11.
101 E.L. Stone to Dr. Mulloy, April 10, 1931, LAC, RG 29, vol. 2823, file 831-1-X444, pt. 1.
102 Sister Superior to Reverend General, March 24, 1924, GNAM, HNDSD, unnumbered document.
103 Dr. Kennedy to Superior General, June 22, 1922, GNAM, HNDSD, Doc. 149.
104 Chronicles, December 1921, p. 146; December 1922, p. 157; December 1923, p. 169; and December 1925, p. 190. Sister Superior to Reverend General, October 30, 1924, unnumbered document, and Sister Superior to Reverend General, December 23, 1905, Doc. 112. All documents in GNAM, HNDSD.
105 Ibid.
106 Reverend General to Sister Superior, March 25, 1928, GNAM, HNDSD, Doc. 171.
107 Dr. Follett to Sarcee Agent Fleetham, April 23, 1915, and Dr. Follett to Dr. Grain, March 2, 1915, LAC, RG 29, vol. 3403, box 229, file 823-1-A772, pt. l.
108 Sarcee Agent Fleetham to Tims, June 29, 1915, GA, Anglican Church, Calgary Indian Missions, Medical Reports, M1356, vol. 6.
109 Secretary of CMS to Tims, February 19, 1897, and Tims to Mr. O'Meara of CMS, March 1, 1897, GA, Calgary Indian Missions, M1356, vol. 2.
110 Sharyn Janes, "Transcultural Nursing and Global Health," in *Essentials of Community-Based Nursing*, ed. Karen Saucier Lundy and Sharyn Janes (Sudbury, On: Jones and Bartlett, 2003), 122-24.
111 Mary Ann Ruffing-Rahal, "The Navajo Experience of Elizabeth Forster, Public Health Nurse," *Nursing History Review* 3 (1995): 173-74.
112 Ibid., 185.
113 Emily Abel and Nancy Reifel, "Interactions between Public Health Nurses and Clients during the 1930s," *Social History of Medicine* 9, 1 (1996): 90. See also Reifel, "American Indian Views of Public Health Nursing," 151-52.
114 Reifel, "American Indian Views," 152.
115 Karen Flint, "Competition, Race, and Professionalization: African Healers and White Medical Practitioners in Natal, South Africa in the Early Twentieth Century," *Social History of Medicine* 14, 2 (2001): 209.
116 McPherson, "Nursing and Colonization," 228-29.
117 Ibid., 240-41.
118 Jane Megarry, diary, n.d., GA, Jane Megarry's Fonds, M4096, vol. 2.
119 Blood Band Council to Scott, May 31, 1927, LAC, RG 29, vol. 2823, file 831-1-X444, pt. 1.
120 Megarry, diary, n.d.
121 E.L. Stone to Dr. Mulloy, April 10, 1931, LAC, RG 29, vol. 2609, file 800-1X444, pt. 1.
122 Megarry, diary, n.d.
123 Reifel, "American Indian View of Public Health Nurses," 146.
124 Miss Murray, "News from the Field," *Letter Leaflet*, August 1910, 302-3.
125 George First Rider, Kainai elder, April 10, 1969, First Nations University of Canada (FNUC), Indian History Film Project (IHFP), IH AA021; Ruffing-Rahal, "The Navajo Experience of Elizabeth Forster," 180.
126 Reifel, "American Indian View of Public Health Nurses," 147-48.
127 Megarry, diary, n.d.

128 Peigan Agent G.H. Wheatley to DIA, August 1899, LAC, RG 10, vol. 1429; Blood Agent J.H. Gooderham to DIA, January 15, 1913, LAC, RG 10, vol. 1540; Bishop of St. Albert to DIA, January 9, 1913; Blood Agent J.H. Gooderham Scott, January 31, 1913; Blood Agent J.H. Gooderham to DIA, March 18, 1913, LAC, RG 10, vol. 1540; Blood Agent J.H. Gooderham to DIA, November 7, 1920, LAC, RG 10, vol. 1541.
129 Reverend Gibbon Stocken to Blackfoot Agent J.H. Gooderham, February 26, 1912, LAC, RG 10, vol. 1153.
130 Ibid.
131 Blood Agent R.N. Wilson to DIA, April 3, 1911, LAC, RG 10, vol. 1540.
132 Ibid., Blood Agent Hyde to DIA, January 15, 1913.
133 Peigan Agent Wilson to DIA, August 1899, LAC, RG 10, vol. 1429.
134 Blood Agent Hyde to DIA, January 15, 1913, LAC, RG 10, vol. 1540.
135 Dr. Kennedy to Superior General, February 19, 1929, GNAM, HNDSD, Doc. 188.

Chapter 6: Taking over the System

1 Kathryn McPherson, "Nursing and Colonization: The Work of Indian Health Service Nurses in Manitoba," in *Women, Health, and Nation: Canada and the United States since 1945*, ed. Georgina Feldberg et al. (Montreal/Kingston: McGill-Queen's University Press, 2003): 238.
2 Cochrane and Area Historical Society, eds., *Big Hill Country: Cochrane and Area* (Cochrane, AB: Cochrane and Area Historical Society, 1977), 92.
3 Memorandum, Scott, March 7, 1910, and Memo from Scott, March 28, 1911, Library and Archives Canada (LAC), RG 10, Department of Indian Affairs, vol. 3957, file 140, pp. 754-61; Brian Titley, *A Narrow Vision: Duncan Campbell Scott and the Administration of Indian Affairs in Canada* (Vancouver: UBC Press, 1986), 24.
4 Mary-Ellen Kelm found similar results in her examination of Aboriginal communities in British Columbia and argues that a pluralistic rather than a hybrid medical system developed. Mary-Ellen Kelm, *Colonizing Bodies: Aboriginal Health and Healing in British Columbia, 1900-1950* (Vancouver: UBC Press, 1998), 153.
5 The professional anthropologists who worked among Aboriginal peoples who lived in the Treaty 7 area during the early twentieth century recorded a range of Aboriginal healing practices but failed to publish this information. Their texts instead evaluate the impact of the state's assimilative programs. The greatest difference between these observers of Plains cultures and later ones is the presence of women among the latter. Until the late 1930s, when Jane Richardson Hanks and Esther Goldfrank conducted fieldwork among the Siksika, anthropologists and ethnographers were predominantly middle-class white men. The presence of white women, and contemporary debates during the 1930s regarding the place and role of birth control in North American society more generally, made issues of childbirth, contraception, and abortion in Aboriginal communities topical concerns.
6 Blood Agency, Dr. Steele to DIA, April 5, 1918, LAC, RG 10, vol. 1541.
7 For examples see Report, Blood Agent Pocklington, June 4, 1890, LAC, RG 10, vol. 3759, file 31949; Monthly Report, Sarcee Agent Lucas, March 12, 1895, LAC, RG 10, vol. 1642; Dr. J.H. Rivers to Blood Agent Wilson, November 14, 1903, Glenbow Archives (GA), Blood Indian Agency Fonds (DIA), M1788, vol. 21.
8 Report, Blood Agent Pocklington, June 4, 1890.

9 Monthly Report, Sarcee Agent Lucas, March 12, 1895; Rivers to Wilson, November 14, 1903.
10 Blood Agent Wilson to Indian Commissioner, April 27, 1905, Blood Letter Books, LAC, RG 10, vol. 1548.
11 Dr. Lafferty to Peigan Agent Wilson, June 26, 1901, LAC, RG 10, vol. 1413.
12 Report, Inspector Wadsworth, July 20, 1900, LAC, RG 10, vol. 3632, file 6326; Canada, *Annual Report of the Department of Indian Affairs for the Year Ended March 31, 1910* (Ottawa: Queen's Printer, 1911), xxiii; Canada, *Annual Report of the Department of Indian Affairs (1913)*, 173; Canada, *Annual Report of the Department of Indian Affairs (1915)*, 70; Report, Peigan Agent Arthur, April 9, 1923, LAC, RG 10, vol. 1425; Canada, *Annual Report of the Department of Indian Affairs (1926)*, 10.
13 Lucien and Jane Richardson Hanks, *Tribe under Trust: A Study of the Blackfoot Reserve of Alberta* (Toronto: University of Toronto Press, 1950), 78.
14 "Field Notes," GA, Lucien M. and Jane Richardson Hanks Fonds, M8458, box 3, file 64, pp. 115-16.
15 Ibid.
16 Ibid.
17 "Field Notes," ibid., box 2, file 37, p. 2.
18 Rufus Goodstriker, Kainai elder, February 14, 1983, First Nations University of Canada (FNUC), Indian History Film Project (IHFP), IH 008.
19 Rufus Goodstriker, Kainai elder, February 14, 1983, FNUC, IHFP, IH 007.
20 Annie Bare Shin Bone, in Flora Zaharia and Leo Fox, eds., *Kitomahkitapiiminnooniksi: Stories from Our Elders* (Edmonton: Donahue House, 1995), 1:12.
21 Mike Mountain Horse, *My People the Bloods* (Calgary: Glenbow-Alberta Institute, 1979), 67-80.
22 Joan Scott-Brown, "Stoney Ethnobotany: An Indication of Cultural Change amongst Stoney Women of Morley Alberta" (master's thesis, University of Calgary, 1977), 148.
23 Blood Agent Dilworth to Dr. Tupper, September 1916, LAC, RG 10, vol. 1541.
24 Blood Agent Dilworth to Scott, June 17, 1916, ibid.
25 Mary-Ellen Kelm, "A Scandalous Procession: Residential Schooling and Re/formation of Aboriginal Bodies, 1900-1950," *Native Studies Review* 11, 2 (1996): 55-57.
26 Peigan Correspondence, Indian Commissioner Graham to Peigan Agent Graham, May 5, 1922, LAC, RG 10, vol. 1425.
27 Ibid.
28 *An Act to Amend the Indian Act*, SC 1914, c. 35, s. 6.
29 Megan Sproule-Jones, "Crusading for the Forgotten: Dr. Peter Bryce, Public Health, and Prairie Native Residential Schools," *Canadian Bulletin of Medical History/Bulletin canadien d'histoire de la médecine* 13, 2 (1996): 218.
30 James Waldram, D. Ann Herring, and T. Kue Young, *Aboriginal Health in Canada: Historical, Cultural, and Epidemiological Perspectives*, 1st ed. (Toronto: University of Toronto Press, 2006), 158-61.
31 Ibid., 160.
32 Maureen Lux, "Perfect Subjects: Race, Tuberculosis, and the Qu'Appelle BCG Vaccine Trial," *Canadian Bulletin of Medical History/Bulletin canadien d'histoire de la médecine* 15 (1998): 284-85; Georgina Feldberg, *Disease and Class: Tuberculosis and the Shaping of Modern North American Society* (New Brunswick, NJ: Rutgers University Press, 1995), 81-124.

33 Canada, *Annual Report of the Department of Indian Affairs for the Year Ended March 31, 1927* (Ottawa: Queen's Printer, 1928), 10-11.
34 Lisa Emmerich, "To Respect and Love and Seek the Ways of White Women: Field Matrons, the Office of Indian Affairs, and Civilization Policy, 1890-1938," (PhD diss., University of Maryland, 1984), 184.
35 Helen Anne English, "The Journals of Helen Anne English, Field Matron on the Little Pine Reserve, 1913-1917," *Saskatchewan History* 45, 2 (1993): 37-42.
36 Canada, *Annual Report (1910)*, 10.
37 Canada, *Annual Report of the Department of Indian Affairs for the Year Ended March 31, 1928* (Ottawa: Queen's Printer, 1929), 9.
38 Scott to Graham, March 23, 1927, LAC, RG 29, National Health and Welfare, vol. 3403, box 4, file 823-1-A772. An examination of the Nakoda pay list for the year 1925-26 revealed twelve births and fourteen deaths. Scott believed that this situation demanded immediate attention.
39 David Gagan and Rosemary Gagan, *For Patients of Moderate Means: A Social History of the Voluntary Public General Hospital in Canada, 1890-1950* (Montreal/Kingston: McGill-Queen's University Press, 2002).
40 Laurie Meijer Drees, "Reserve Hospitals and Medical Officers: Health Care and Indian Peoples in Southern Alberta," *Prairie Forum* 21, 2 (1996): 158.
41 Ibid., 165. Cardston was chosen as the new site because it was a more convenient location and closer to the agency.
42 Ibid., 167-69.
43 Report, A.S. Williams to Dr. McGill, December 6, 1935, GA, Harold Wigmore and Emma Griffis McGill Fonds, M742, vol. 36.
44 "Old Anglican Boarding School Now Sanatorium," *Calgary Herald*, November 17, 1921.
45 Report, A.S. Williams to Dr. McGill, December 6, 1935.
46 Biographical Sketch, GA, Harold Wigmore and Emma Griffis McGill Fonds, M742.
47 Waldram, Herring, and Young, *Aboriginal Health in Canada*, 160.
48 Ibid., 161.
49 Ibid., 165. In 1944 the federal government established a new Department of National Health and Welfare. The following year, Indian and Northern Health Services was incorporated into that department. In 1949, Indian Affairs became part of the Department of Citizenship and Immigration, where it stayed until 1966, when Indian Affairs was transferred to the newly created Department of Indian Affairs and Northern Development (DIAND).
50 Patricia Roome, "From One Whose Home Is among the Indians: Henrietta Muir Edwards and Aboriginal Peoples," in *Unsettled Pasts: Reconceiving the West through Women's History*, ed. Sarah Carter et al. (Calgary: University of Calgary Press, 2005), 62.
51 Ibid.
52 Waldram, Herring, and Young, *Aboriginal Health in Canada*, 156-65.
53 Report, Peigan Agent Gunn, August 5, 1916, LAC, RG 10, vol. 1425.
54 Blackfoot Agent Gooderham to W.M. Graham, November 19, 1928, LAC, RG 29, vol. 2919, file 851-1-A772, pt. 1.
55 Maureen Lux, *Medicine That Walks: Disease, Medicine, and Canadian Plains Native People, 1880-1940* (Toronto: University of Toronto Press, 2001), 168-70. See also Canada, *Annual Report of the Department of Indian Affairs for the Year Ended March 31, 1907* (Ottawa: Queen's

Printer, 1908), 276; Monthly Reports for the Blood Hospital, 1901 to 1924, LAC, RG 10, vol. 1540.
56 Lux, *Medicine That Walks*, 170. Herbs that caused individuals to cough up phlegm and aroma therapy to sooth sore throats.
57 John Hellson and Morgan Gadd, *Ethnobotany of the Blackfoot Indians* (Ottawa: National Museums of Canada, 1974), 74.
58 Peigan Correspondence, Indian Commissioner to Peigan Agent Graham, May 5, 1922, LAC, RG 10, vol. 1425.
59 Canada, *Annual Report of the Department of Indian Affairs for the Year Ended June 30, 1904* (Ottawa: Queen's Printer, 1905), xxvii.
60 Peigan Agent Arthur to Scott, June 7, 1923, LAC, RG 29, vol. 2823, file 831-1-A433.
61 Sarcee Agent Fleetham to Tims, April 16, 1915, and J.D. McLean to Tims, April 22, 1915, GA, Anglican Church, Calgary Indian Missions, Medical Reports, M1356, vol. 6; J.D. McLean to Dr. Follett, April 23, 1915, LAC, RG 29, vol. 3403, box 229, file 823-1-A772.
62 Sarcee Agent Fleetham to Tims, April 16 and 19, 1915, and Sarcee Agent Fleetham to Scott, November 2, 1916, LAC, RG 29, vol. 3403, box 229, file 823-1-A772.
63 Ibid.
64 Ibid.
65 Scott to Pringle, April 28, 1927, LAC, RG 29, vol. 3402, file 823-1-A772.
66 Request for Classification of New Position, May 2, 1927, ibid.
67 Canada, *Annual Report of the Department of Indian Affairs for the Year Ended March 31, 1929* (Ottawa: Queen's Printer, 1930), 13.
68 Lux, *Medicine That Walks*, 168-70.
69 Judith Leavitt and Ronald Numbers, "Sickness and Health in America: An Overview," in *Sickness and Health in America*, ed. Judith Leavitt and Ronald Numbers (Madison: University of Wisconsin Press, 1997), 3-10.
70 Richardson and Richardson, *Tribe under Trust*, 50; see also Lux, *Medicine That Walks*, 163.
71 Report, Dr. J.J. Wall, "Trachoma among the Indians of Western Canada," n.d., LAC, RG 29, vol. 288, file 402-7-2.
72 Nurse Agnes Hucomb, December 31, 1916. Nurse Maude Hill, January 31, February 31, April 31, May 31, October 31, and December 31, 1917; January 31, February 28, and March 31, 1918. Nurse's Report, April 1919 and May 1919. Nurse Isabel Reinhardt, April 1919. Nurse Jessie Underhill, January 14, 1920. Nurse Reinhardt, January 8, 1921. In GA, Anglican Church, Calgary Indian Missions, Medical Reports, M1356, vol. 6.
73 Nurse Maude Hill, January 31; Dr. MacNab to Reverend Tims, March 10, 1917. In GA, Anglican Church, Calgary Indian Missions, Medical Reports, M1356, vol. 6.
74 Dr. Kennedy to Blood Agent Ostrauder, January 25, 1926, Grey Nuns Archives, Montreal (GNAM), Hôpital Notre-Dame-des-Sept-Douleurs/Stand Off, Blood Reserve, Alberta, L049 (HNDSD), Doc. 170.
75 Ibid.
76 Dr. Kennedy to Reverend Mother, August 11, 1924, ibid., Doc. 154; Dr. Kennedy to DIA, June 17, 1922, ibid., Doc. 150.
77 Dr. Stone to Dr. Mulloy, April 10, 1931, LAC, RG 29, vol. 2609, file 800-1-X444, pt. 1.
78 Dr. Kennedy to Reverend Mother, August 11, 1924.
79 Dr. Kennedy to DIA, June 17, 1922.
80 Report Regarding the Blackfoot Hospital, February 18, 1926, LAC, RG 29, vol. 2592, file 800-1-0443.

81 Sister Superior to Blood Agent Ostrauder, May 14, 1924, LAC, RG 10, vol. 1542.
82 Nurse's report for September 1917 and July 1917, GA, Anglican Church, Calgary Indian Missions, Medical Reports, M1356, vol. 6.
83 S. Stuart, Assistant Secretary DIA, to Bishop McNally, October 30, 1915, GNAM, HNDSD, Doc. 142.
84 Dr. Alan Kennedy to Superior *General,* March 23, 1927, ibid., Doc. 159.
85 Kathryn McPherson, *Bedside Matters: The Transformation of Canadian Nursing, 1900-1990* (Toronto: Oxford University Press, 1996), 74-114.
86 Father Renaud to DIA, December 2, 1931, LAC, RG 29, vol. 2609, file 800-1-X444, pt. 1.
87 Sister Superior to Blood Agent Pugh, February 11, 1931, GNAM, HNDSD, Doc. 181.
88 David Williams, Archbishop of Huron, Chairman of the CMS to Scott, March 20, 1928, General Synod Archives (GSA), Anglican Church of Canada (ACC), Missionary Society Papers (MSP), GS 75-103, box 28.
89 Reverend Sherman, Bishop of Calgary, to Scott, April 30, 1927, LAC, RG 29, vol. 2823, file 831-1-x444, pt. 1.
90 Petition to Scott, May 31, 1927, ibid.
91 Blood Agent Pugh to Scott, May 18, 1927, ibid.
92 Report, J.K. Mulloy, March 17, 1930, LAC, RG 29, vol. 2609, file 800-1-x444, pt. 1; Sister Superior to Father Guy, February 17, 1927, LAC, RG 29, vol. 2823, file 831-1-x444, pt. 1; Sister Superior to Scott, March 24, 1927, GNAM, HNDSD, Doc. 174.
93 Scott to Sister Superior, March 22, 1928, LAC, RG 29, vol. 2609, file 800-1-x444; Scott to Sister Superior, March 22, 1927, GNAM, HNDSD, Doc. 14.1.
94 Reverend General to Bishop of Calgary, April 10, 1928, GNAM, HNDSD, Doc. 14.3.
95 Bishop of Calgary to Reverend General, April 10, 1928, ibid., Doc. 176.
96 Reverend General to Sister Superior, June 20, 1928, ibid., Doc. 180.
97 McGill to Reverend General, June 13, 1931, GA, Harold McGill Fonds, M742, vol. 36.
98 McGill to Reverend General, May 18, 1934, ibid.
99 Reverend General to Bishop of Calgary, May 28, 1934, GNAM, HNDSD, Doc. 15.1.
100 McCallum, M.G. "The Alberta Department of Public Health," in *The Federal and Provincial Health Services in Canada,* ed. R.D. Defries 2nd ed. (Ottawa: Canadian Public Health Association, 1962), 110.
101 Sharon Richardson, "Frontier Health Care: Alberta's District and Municipal Nursing Services, 1919 to 1976," *Alberta History* 46, 1 (1998): 3.
102 Irene Stewart, ed., *These Were Our Yesterdays: A History of District Nursing in Alberta* (Calgary: Friesen Printers, 1979), 11.
103 Sharon Richardson, "Alberta's Provincial Travelling Clinic, 1924-42," *Canadian Bulletin of Medical History/Bulletin canadien d'histoire de la médecine* 19 (2002): 246.
104 Ibid., 248.
105 Canada, *Sixth Census of Canada, 1921* (Ottawa: King's Printer, 1924), 350-55.
106 Ibid., 182-201.
107 Stewart, "These Were Our Yesterdays," 64.
108 Richardson, "Alberta's Provincial Travelling Clinic," 254.
109 Ibid., 257.
110 Lux, *Medicine That Walks,* 138-39.
111 Pamela Margaret White, "Restructuring the Domestic Sphere: Prairie Indian Women on Reserves – Image, Ideology, and State Policy, 1880-1930" (PhD diss., McGill University, 1987), 234.

112 Canada, *Annual Report of the Department of Indian Affairs for the Year Ended March 31, 1924* (Ottawa: Queen's Printer, 1925), 12.
113 Canada, *Annual Report of the Department of Indian Affairs for the Year Ended March 31, 1927* (Ottawa: Queen's Printer, 1928), 11.
114 Ibid., 10-11.
115 Neil Sutherland, *Children in English-Canadian Society: Framing the Twentieth-Century Consensus* (Waterloo: Wilfred Laurier University Press, 1978 [2000]), 188-90.
116 Canada, *Annual Report of the Department of Indian Affairs for the Year Ended June 30, 1903* (Ottawa: Queen's Printer, 1904), xxvii.
117 Canada, *Annual Report for the Department of Indian Affairs for the Year Ended March 31, 1909* (Ottawa: Queen's Printer, 1910), xxiii.
118 Adele Perry, "From the Hot-Bed of Vice to the Good and Well-Ordered Christian Home: First Nations' Housing and Reform in Nineteenth-Century British Columbia," *Ethnohistory* 50, 4 (2003): 587-610.
119 John Lutz, "Relating to the Country: The Lekwammen and the Extension of European Settlement," in *Beyond the City Limits: Rural History in British Columbia*, ed. R.W. Sandwell (Vancouver: UBC Press, 1999), 27.
120 Report, Blackfoot Agent Gooderham, February 18, 1926, LAC, RG 10, vol. 4093, file 600-178.
121 Annmarie Adams, *Architecture in the Family Way: Doctors, Houses, and Women, 1870-1900* (Montreal/Kingston: McGill-Queen's University Press, 1996), 103.
122 Indian Commissioner to Peigan Agent Wilson, February 16, 1898, LAC, RG 10, vol. 1413; Peigan Agent Graham to Graham, May 22, 1922, LAC, RG 10, vol. 1425; Blackfoot Agent Gooderham to Scott, June 29, 1926, LAC, RG 10, vol. 4093, file 600-178; Canada, *Annual Report of the Department of Indian Affairs for the Year Ended March 31, 1910* (Ottawa: Queen's Printer, 1911), xxii; Canada, *Annual Report of the Department of Indian Affairs for the Year Ended March 31, 1911* (Ottawa: Queen's Printer, 1912), xxii; Canada, *Annual Report (1926)*, 11; Canada, *Annual Report of the Department of Indian Affairs for the Year Ended March 31, 1928* (Ottawa: Queen's Printer, 1929), 9; Canada, *Annual Report of the Department of Indian Affairs for the Year Ended March 31, 1932* (Ottawa: Queen's Printer, 1933), 8.
123 Scott to Morley Agent Pringle, March 7, 1927, and Scott to Bennett, March 7, 1927, LAC, RG 29, vol. 3403, box 229, file 823-1-A772.
124 Report, Stoney Agent Pringle, March 15, 1927, LAC, RG 29, vol. 3403, box 229, file 823-1-A772.
125 Ibid.
126 Ibid., May 14, 1925.
127 Ibid., Stoney Agent Pringle to Scott, March 30, 1927.
128 Nadine Kozak, "Advice and Rural Prairie Realities: National and Prairie Scientific Motherhood Advice, 1920-29," in *Unsettled Pasts: Reconceiving the West through Women's History*, ed. Carter et al., 180.
129 Dianne Dodd, "Advice to Parents: The Blue Books, Helen MacMurchy, MD, and the Federal Department of Health, 1920-34," *Canadian Bulletin of Medical History/Bulletin canadien d'histoire de la médecine* 8, 1 (1991): 204.
130 Canada, *Annual Report (1896)*, 202.
131 Report, Peigan Agent Graham, June 8, 1922, LAC, RG 10, vol. 1425.
132 Maude Hill, Medical Reports, April 1917 and September 1917, GA, Anglican Church, Calgary Indian Missions, M1356, vol. 6; Report, Stoney Agent Pringle, March 15, 1927,

and Scott to Bennett, March 23, 1927, LAC, RG 29, vol. 3403, box 229, file 823-1-A772; Blood Agent Dilworth to Scott, June 17, 1916, LAC, RG 10, vol. 1541; Canada, *Annual Report (1896)*, 202.
133 Scott to Blackfoot Agent Gooderham, March 9, 1926, LAC, RG 10, vol. 4093, file 600-178.
134 Report, Blackfoot Agent Gooderham, February 18, 1926, ibid.
135 Scott to Blackfoot Agent Gooderham, March 9, 1926.
136 Scott to R.B. Bennett, March 7, 1927, LAC, RG 29, vol. 3403, box 229, file 823-1-A772.
137 Hill, Medical Reports, May 1917, April 1917, February 1917, and September 1917.
138 Ibid., February 1917.
139 Ibid., July 1917.
140 Ibid., February 1917.
141 Ibid., December 1917.
142 Canada, *Annual Report of the Department of Indian Affairs for the Year Ended March 31, 1913* (Ottawa: Queen's Printer, 1914), 169.
143 Canada, *Annual Report of the Department of Indian Affairs for the Year Ended March 31, 1916* (Ottawa: Queen's Printer, 1917), 77.
144 Blackfoot Agent Gooderham to Scott, March 30, 1926, LAC, RG 10, vol. 4093, file 600-178.
145 Ibid.
146 Judge's Comment Card for Baby Show at the Blackfoot Hospital, n.d., ibid.
147 Gerald Thomson, "A Baby Show Means Work in the Hardest Sense: The Better Baby Contests of the Vancouver and New Westminster Local Councils of Women, 1913-1929," *BC Studies*, no. 128 (Winter 2000-01): 35.
148 Newspaper clipping, *Winnipeg Free Press*, April 1, 1933, LAC, RG 10, vol. 4093, file 600-178.
149 Ibid.
150 Indian Commissioner to Blood Agent J.T. Faunt, September 4, 1924; Annie Brandon to Blood Agent J.T. Faunt, October 28, 1924; and Blood Agent J.T. Faunt to Miss Brandon, November 19, 1924, GA, Blood Indian Agency Fonds, Correspondence, M1788, vol. 18.
151 Brandon to Faunt, October 28, 1924, ibid.
152 Canada, *Annual Report (1896)*, 156; Canada, *Annual Report (1903)*, xxvii; Canada, *Annual Report (1924)*, 12.
153 Mariana Valverde, *The Age of Light, Soap, Water: Moral Reform in English Canada, 1885-1925* (Toronto: McClelland and Stewart, 1991), 129-54. Similarities are apparent regarding middle-class descriptions of Aboriginal housing on reserves and working-class slums in urban areas. According to Valverde, "the evil deeds taking place in the secret darkness of the slum were legion: prostitution, alcoholism, thriftlessness, child neglect, gambling, stealing, lack of hygiene, irreligion, contagious disease, swearing, bad eating habits, 'the love of finery,' and Sabbath-breaking," 134.
154 Ibid., 49.
155 Canada, *Annual Report (1926)*, 10; Canada, *Annual Report (1927)*, 10; Canada, *Annual Report (1928)*, 8-9.

Chapter 7: The Snake and the Butterfly

1 Dianne Dodd, "Helen MacMurchy: Popular Midwifery and Maternity Services for Canadian Pioneer Women," in *Caring and Curing: Historical Perspectives on Women and*

Healing in Canada, ed. Dianne Dodd and Deborah Gorham (Ottawa: University of Ottawa Press, 1994), 135.
2 Patricia Jasen, "Race, Culture, and the Colonization of Childbirth in Northern Canada," *Social History of Medicine* 10, 3 (1997): 392.
3 Betty-Anne Daviss, "Heeding Warnings from the Canary, the Whale, and the Inuit: A Framework for Analyzing Competing Types of Knowledge about Childbirth," in *Childbirth and Authoritative Knowledge: Cross-Cultural Perspectives,* ed. Robbie Davis-Floyd and Carolyn Sargent (Berkeley: University of California Press, 1997), 441-73; John O'Neil and Patricia Kaufert, "Irniktakpunga! Sex Determination and the Inuit Struggle for Birthing Rights in Northern Canada," in *Conceiving the New World Order: The Global Politics of Reproduction,* ed. Faye Ginsburg and Rayna Rapp (Berkeley: University of California Press, 1995), 59-73. See also Lynn Bourgeault, *Push! The Struggle for Midwifery in Ontario* (Montreal/Kingston: McGill-Queen's University Press, 2006).
4 Bourgeault, *Push!* See also Margaret MacDonald, *Work in the Field of Birth: Midwifery Narratives of Nature, Tradition, and Home* (Nashville, TN: Vanderbilt University Press, 2007), and Sheryl Nestel, *Obstructed Labour: Race and Gender in the Re-emergence of Midwifery* (Vancouver: UBC Press, 2006).
5 An exception to this rule is the brief discussion of childbirth practices among northwestern Plains peoples that Maureen Lux includes in *Medicine That Walks: Disease, Medicine, and Canadian Plains Native People* (Toronto: University of Toronto Press, 2001).
6 Dena Carroll and Cecilia Benoit, "Aboriginal Midwifery in Canada: Merging Traditional Practices and Modern Science," in *Reconceiving Midwifery,* ed. Ivy Bourgeault, Cecilia Benoit, and Robbie Davis-Floyd, eds. (Montreal/Kingston: McGill-Queen's University Press, 2004), 265.
7 Pamela White, "Restructuring the Domestic Sphere: Prairie Indian Women on Reserves – Image, Ideology, and State Policy, 1880-1930" (PhD diss., McGill University, 1987), 237.
8 Ibid., 239.
9 Cynthia Comacchio, *"Nations Are Built of Babies": Saving Ontario's Mothers and Children, 1900-1940* (Montreal/Kingston: McGill Queen's University Press, 1993), 65-67.
10 Sharon Richardson, "Frontier Health Care: Alberta's District and Municipal Nursing Services, 1919 to 1976." *Alberta History* 46, 1 (1998): 2-3.
11 Ibid., 3.
12 Wendy Mitchinson, *Giving Birth in Canada, 1900-1950* (Toronto: University of Toronto Press, 2002), 160. See also Jasen, "Race, Culture, and the Colonization of Childbirth in Northern Canada," 383-400.
13 David Gagan and Rosemary Gagan, *For Patients of Moderate Means: A Social History of the Voluntary Public General Hospital in Canada, 1890-1950* (Montreal/Kingston: McGill-Queen's University Press, 2002), 3.
14 Dr. Kennedy to Blood Agent Faunt, January 25, 1926, Grey Nuns Archives, Montreal (GNAM), Hôpital Notre-Dame-des-Sept-Douleurs/Stand Off, Blood Reserve, Alberta, L049 (hereafter HNDSD), Doc. 170.
15 Mitchinson, *Giving Birth in Canada,* 173-78.
16 Comacchio, *Nations Are Built of Babies.*
17 Lux, *Medicine That Walks,* 97.
18 Flora Zaharia and Leo Fox, ed., *Kitomahkitapiiminnooniksi: Stories from Our Elders,* vol. 1-3 (Edmonton: Donahue House, 1995).
19 Mitchinson, *Giving Birth in Canada,* 184, 190-230.

20 "The Hospital," unpublished article, December 1955, Glenbow Archives (GA), George H. Gooderham Fonds, M4738, box 3.
21 "Field Notes," GA, Lucien M. and Jane Richardson Hanks Fonds, M8458, box 3, file 64, p. 1.
22 Blood Hospital Monthly Reports, October 1923 to November 1924, Library and Archives Canada (LAC), RG 10, Department of Indian Affairs, vol. 1540.
23 Suzanne Olivier, "Historique," p. 2; and Reverend General to Bishop of Calgary, April 29, 1916, GNAM, HNDSD, Doc. 143.
24 Marta Danylewycz, *Taking the Veil: An Alternative to Marriage, Motherhood, and Spinsterhood in Quebec, 1840-1920* (Toronto: McClelland and Stewart, 1987), 20; see also Laura Ettinger, "Mission to Mothers: Nuns, Latino Families, and the Founding of Santa Fe's Catholic Maternity Institute," in *Women, Health, and Nation: Canada and the United States since 1945*, ed. Georgina Feldberg et al. (Montreal/Kingston: McGill-Queen's University Press, 2003), 144-60.
25 Blood Agent Hyde to DIA, February 25, 1913, LAC, RG 10, 1542.
26 Blood Agent Hyde to DIA, November 5, 1912, and February 25, 1913, and J.D. McLean to Blood Agent Hyde, December 16, 1912, ibid; Bishop of St. Albert to Reverend General, January 12, 1913, GNAM, HNDSD, Doc. 125.
27 Reverend General to Bishop of St. Albert, January 15, 1913, unnumbered document; Bishop of St. Albert to Reverend General, January 23, 1913 Doc. 129; Reverend General to Bishop of St. Albert, January 30, 1913, Doc. 129; S. Stuart, Assistant Deputy and Secretary of Indian Affairs, to Bishop of Calgary, 30 October 1915, Doc. 142; Reverend General to Bishop of Calgary, October 28, 1916, Doc. 145; Reverend General to Bishop of Calgary, April 29, 1916, Doc. 142. All in GNAM, HNDSD.
28 Suzanne Olivier, "Historique," 2, and Reverend General to Bishop of Calgary, April 29, 1916, Doc. 143, in GNAM, HNDSD.
29 Reverend General to Bishop of Calgary, April 29, 1916, Doc. 142, GNAM, HNDSD.
30 Bishop of St. Albert to Reverend General, January 23, 1913, unnumbered document, GNAM, HNDSD.
31 Bishop of St. Albert to Reverend General, January 12, 1913, Doc. 125, GNAM, HNDSD.
32 Reverend General to Bishop of Calgary, October 28, 1916, Doc. 145, GNAM, HNDSD.
33 Ettinger, "Mission to Mothers," 148.
34 Ibid., 144-60.
35 "Field Notes," GA, Lucien M. and Jane Richardson Hanks Fonds, M8458, box 3, file 64, p. 175.
36 "Field Notes," GA, Esther Goldfrank Fonds, M243, 43.
37 Carroll and Benoit, "Aboriginal Midwifery in Canada," 267-68.
38 Diamond Jenness, *The Sarcee Indians of Alberta* (Ottawa: National Museum of Canada, 1938), 26-27.
39 Ibid., 26.
40 Goldfrank's field notes do not indicate what the pain killer was in part because anthropologists were concerned with chronicling the social and cultural aspects of northwestern Plains cultures and not the medicinal qualities of local plant life.
41 Beverly Hungry Wolf, *The Ways of My Grandmothers* (New York: William Morrow, 1980), 191-94.
42 Agnes Red Crow, in Zaharia and Fox, eds., *Kitomahkitapiiminnooniksi*, 1:102.
43 Frank Eagle Tail Feathers, in ibid., 2:15.

44 Allan Shade, in ibid., 2:53.
45 Zaharia and Fox, eds., *Kitomahkitapiiminnooniksi*, vols. 1-3.
46 Ibid.
47 Violet was a graduate of the Blackfoot residential school. This experience may have affected her choice of location for the birth of her first baby.
48 "Field Notes," GA, Esther Goldfrank Fonds, M243, 380-81.
49 Ibid.
50 Angus McLaren, "Keep Your Seats and Face Facts: Western Canadian Women's Discussion of Birth Control in the 1920s," *Canadian Bulletin of Medical History/Bulletin canadien d'histoire de la médecine* 8, 2 (1991): 192.
51 Mary Bishop, "Vivian Dowding: Birth Control Activist," in *Rethinking Canada: The Promise of Women's History*, ed. Veronica Strong-Boag and Anita Fellman (Toronto: Copp Clark Pitman, 1986), 201.
52 Notes on the Blackfoot, Blood, and Peigan Indians, vol. 2, April 29, 1911, p. 321, GA, David C. Duvall Fonds.
53 Ibid.
54 Ibid.
55 "Field Notes," GA, Esther Goldfrank Fonds, M243, 372.
56 Ibid.
57 Ibid.
58 "Field Notes," GA, Claude Everett Schaeffer Fonds, M1100, vol. 137. The rattlesnake is said to have no friends, and all beings fear it. That is why it is used. An otter is fond of the water, and is also feared by people. It moves as quickly as a snake in the water. Both spirits are very powerful.
59 Ibid.
60 Ibid. Takes Gun On Top also helped women who miscarried, but the nature of that assistance is not indicated in the field notes.
61 Ibid.
62 Angus McLaren, *Reproductive Rituals: The Perception of Fertility in England from the Sixteenth to the Nineteenth Century* (London: Methuen, 1984), 5.
63 "Field Notes," GA, Claude Everett Schaeffer Fonds, M1100, vol. 137.
64 Ibid.
65 Hungry Wolf, *The Ways of My Grandmothers*, 203.
66 GA, Esther Goldfrank Fonds, M243, 278.
67 "Field Notes," GA, Claude Everett Schaeffer Fonds, M1100, vol. 137.
68 Ibid.
69 George First Rider, Kainai elder, March 27, 1969, First Nations University of Canada (FNUC), Indian History Film Project (IHFP), IH AA079.
70 John Hellson and Morgan Gadd, *Ethnobotany of the Blackfoot Indians* (Ottawa: National Museums of Canada, 1974), 57.
71 Ibid.
72 Ibid., 58.
73 Mary-Ellen Kelm, *Colonizing Bodies: Aboriginal Health and Healing in British Columbia, 1900-1950* (Vancouver: UBC Press, 1998), 153-72.
74 Lux, *Medicine That Walks*, 77; Joan Scott-Brown, "Stoney Ethnobotany: An Indication of Cultural Change amongst Stoney Women of Morley Alberta" (master's thesis, University of Calgary, 1977), 148.

Conclusion

1 Rev. E.F. Wilson, "Report on the Sarcee Indians," *Report of the British Association for the Advancement of Science* 58 (1888): 242-55 (emphasis in original). Wilson was a clergyman for the Anglican Church, a teacher, an ethnologist, and an author.
2 Andrea Smith, *Conquest: Sexual Violence and American Indian Genocide* (Cambridge: South End, 2005), 9.

Bibliography

ARCHIVAL COLLECTIONS

Alexander Galt Archives (AGA)

Blood Indian Agency Papers
Alexander Johnston Papers

City of Edmonton Archives (CEA)

Edna Kells Manuscripts, MS10

First Nations University of Canada (FNUC)

Indian History Film Projects (IHFP)
    Marion Carrier, Cree elder, IH 017
    Jack Crow, Piikani elder, IH 231
    George First Rider, Kainai elder, IH AA021, IH AA079
    Rufus Goodstriker, Kainai elder, IH 007, IH 008

General Synod Archives (GSA), Anglican Church of Canada (ACC)

Missionary Society Papers (MSP)

Glenbow Archives (GA)

Anglican Church, Calgary Indian Missions
Anglican Mission Workers, Letters
Blackfoot Indian Agency Fonds (DIA)
Blood Indian Agency Fonds (DIA)

F.C Cornish Fonds
David C. Duvall Fonds
Esther Goldfrank Fonds
George H. Gooderham Family Fonds
Lucien M. and Jane Richardson Hanks Fonds
Oscar Lewis Fonds
Peigan Indian Agency Fonds (DIA)
McDougall Family Fonds
Jane Megarry Fonds
Sarcee Indian Agency Fonds (DIA)
Claude Everett Schaeffer Fonds
Marie Rose Smith Fonds
Stoney Indian Agency Fonds (DIA)
Alice Turner Fonds
Harold Wigmore and Emma Griffis McGill Fonds

Grey Nun Archives, Montreal (GNAM)

Hôpital Notre-Dame-des-Sept-Douleurs (HNDSD), Stand Off and Cardston, Blood Reserve, Alberta, L049

Library and Archives Canada (LAC)

Canadian Tuberculosis Association
Department of Indian Affairs, RG 10
Wilfred Laurier Papers
National Health and Welfare, RG 29
Royal Canadian Mounted Police, RG 18

Provincial Archives of Alberta (PAA)

Blood Hospital Registers

Saskatchewan Archives Board (SAB)

Pioneer Questionnaires, File 8, Health
Regina Women's Canadian Club Convention, R-176, I22
Effie Storer Papers

United Church of Canada (UCC), Victoria College Archives (VCA)

Marchmont Ing Papers
K. Margaret Laing, Biographical Outline
John Maclean Papers
Methodist Church Missionary Society, Foreign Department, T.E.E Shore Papers

University of Calgary, Special Collections (UCSC)

Anglican Church of Canada (ACC), Calgary Diocese (CD)

Bibliography

NEWSPAPERS AND MAGAZINES

Calgary Herald
Christian Guardian
Letter Leaflet
Maclean's Magazine
Medicine Hat News
Missionary Outlook

PUBLISHED PRIMARY SOURCES

Adam, François. "Duhamel." *Alberta Folklore Quarterly* 1, 1 (1945): 14-15.
Ames, Herbert Brown. *The City Below the Hill.* Toronto: University of Toronto Press, 1972 [1897].
Bryce, P.H. *Report on the Indian Schools of Manitoba and the North West Territories.* Ottawa: Government Printing Bureau, 1907.
Canada. *Census of Canada, 1880-81.* Vol. 1. Ottawa: Maclean, Roger, 1882.
–. *Census of Canada, 1901.* Ottawa: King's Printer, 1903.
–. *Census of Canada, 1921.* Ottawa: King's Printer, 1924.
–. *Census of Canada, 1931.* Ottawa: King's Printer, 1936.
–. *Census of the North-West Provinces, 1906.* Ottawa: King's Printer, 1907.
English, Helen Anne. "The Journals of Helen Anne English, Field Matron on the Little Pine Reserve, 1913-1917." *Saskatchewan History* 45, 2 (1993): 37-42.
Frog Lake Community Club. *Land of Red and White.* Heinsburg, AB: Frog Lake Community Club, 1977.
Goddard, Pliny Earle. "Sarsi Texts." *University of California Publications in American Archaeology and Ethnology* 11, 3 (1915): 189-277.
Grinnell, George Bird. *Blackfoot Lodge Tales: The Story of a Prairie People.* Lincoln: University of Nebraska Press, 1962 [1892].
Hanks, Lucien, and Jane Richardson. *Tribe under Trust: A Study of the Blackfoot Reserve of Alberta.* Toronto: University of Toronto Press, 1950.
Hopkins, Monica. *Letters from a Lady Rancher.* Halifax: Formac Publishing, 1982.
Jenness, Diamond. *The Sarcee Indians of Alberta.* Ottawa: National Museum of Canada, 1938.
Long, W.H., ed. *Fort Pelly Journal of Daily Occurrences, 1863.* Regina: Regina Archaeological Society, 1987.
Maclean, John. "Blackfoot Medical Priesthood." *Medicine Hat News,* October 21, 1909.
–. *Canadian Savage Folk: The Native Tribes of Canada.* Toronto: William Briggs, 1896.
–. *H.B. Steinhauer: His Work among the Cree Indians of the Western Canadian Plains.* Toronto: William Briggs, n.d.
–. *The Indians of Canada: Their Manners and Customs.* Toronto: William Briggs, 1892.
–. *McDougall of Alberta.* Toronto: Ryerson, 1927.
–. *Vanguards of Canada.* Toronto: Missionary Society of the Methodist Church, 1918.
MacMurchy, Helen. *Maternal Mortality in Canada.* Ottawa: Department of Health, 1928.
McClintock, Walter. *The Old North Trail: Life, Legends and Religion of the Blackfoot Indians.* Lincoln: University of Nebraska Press, 1999 [1910].
McDougall, Annie. "Pioneer Life in the 1870s." *Alberta History* 46, 2 (1998): 25-27.

Moosomin: Century One Town and Country. Altona, MB: D.W. Friesen, 1981.
Morris, Alexander. *The Treaties of Canada with the Indians.* Toronto: Prospero Books, 2000 [1880].
Nevitt, R.B. *A Winter at Fort Macleod.* Edited by Hugh Dempsey. Calgary: Glenbow-Alberta Institute, 1974.
Ormsby, Margaret, ed. *A Pioneer Gentlewoman in British Columbia: The Recollections of Susan Allison.* Vancouver: UBC Press, 1976.
Preston, Emmy, ed. *Pioneers of Grandview District.* Steinbach, MB: Carillon Press, 1976.
Price, Elizabeth Bailey. "Pioneers of the Foothills." *MacLean's Magazine,* July 1, 1927, 83-85.
Schultz, James. *Blackfeet Tales of Glacier National Park.* Helena, MO: Riverbend Publishing, 2002 [1916].
–. *My Life as an Indian.* Mineola, NY: Dover Publications, 1997 [1907].
Spry, Irene, ed. *The Palliser Expedition: An Account of John Palliser's British North American Expedition, 1857-1860.* Toronto: Macmillan, 1963.
Stocken, H.W. Gibbon. *Among the Blackfoot and the Sarcee.* Edited by Hugh Dempsey. Calgary: Glenbow Museum, 1987.
Wilson, E.F., Rev. "Report on the Sarcee Indians." *Report of the British Association for the Advancement of Science* 58 (1888): 242-55.
Wissler, Clark. *Social Organization and Ritualistic Ceremonies of the Blackfoot Indians.* New York: AMS Press, 1912.
–. "The Sun Dance of the Blackfoot Indians." In *A Blackfoot Source Book: Papers by Clark Wissler,* ed. David Hurst Thomas. New York: Garland, 1986.
Wissler, Clark, and D.C. Duvall. *Mythology of the Blackfoot Indians.* Lincoln: University of Nebraska Press, 1995 [1908].

Secondary Sources

Abel, Emily, and Nancy Reifel. "Interactions between Public Health Nurses and Clients during the 1930s." *Social History of Medicine* 9, 1 (1996): 89-108.
Adams, Annmarie. *Architecture in the Family Way: Doctors, Houses, and Women, 1870-1900.* Montreal/Kingston: McGill-Queen's University Press, 1996.
Albers, Patricia. "Introduction: New Perspectives on Plains Indian Women." In *The Hidden Half: Studies of Plains Indian Women,* ed. Patricia Albers and Beatrice Medicine, 1-28. Lanham, MD: University Press of America, 1983.
Anderson, Raoul R. "Alberta Stoney (Assiniboine) Origins and Adaptations: A Case for Reappraisal." *Ethnohistory* 17, 1 (1970): 49-61.
Angel, Michael. *Preserving the Sacred: Historical Perspectives on the Ojibwa Midewiwin.* Winnipeg: University of Manitoba Press, 2002.
Archer, S.A., ed. *A Heroine of the North: Memoirs of Charlotte Selina Bompas, 1830-1917.* London: Society for Promoting Christian Knowledge, 1929.
Arnold, David. *Colonizing the Body: State Medicine and Epidemic Disease in Nineteenth-Century India.* Berkeley: University of California Press, 1993.
Backhouse, Constance. "Nineteenth-Century Canadian Prostitution Law: Reflection of a Discriminatory Society." *Social History/Histoire sociale* 18, 36 (1985): 387-423.
Bantjes, Rod. *Improved Earth: Prairie Space as Modern Artefact, 1869-1944.* Toronto: University of Toronto Press, 2005.

Barman, Jean. "Aboriginal Women on the Streets of Victoria: Rethinking Transgressive Sexuality during the Colonial Encounter." In *Contact Zones: Aboriginal and Settler Women in Canada's Colonial Past,* ed. Katie Pickles and Myra Rutherdale, 205-27. Vancouver: UBC Press, 2005.

Bastien, Betty. *Blackfoot Ways of Knowing: The Worldview of the Siksikaitsitapi.* Calgary: University of Calgary Press, 2004.

Biggs, Leslie. "Rethinking the History of Midwifery in Canada." In *Reconceiving Midwifery,* ed. Ivy Lynn Bourgeault, Cecilia Benoit, and Robbi Davis-Floyd, 17-45. Montreal/Kingston: McGill-Queen's University Press, 2004.

Binnema, Theodore. *Common and Contested Ground: A Human and Environmental History of the Northwestern Plains.* Norman: University of Oklahoma Press, 2001.

Bishop, Mary. "Vivian Dowding: Birth Control Activist." In *Rethinking Canada: The Promise of Women's History,* ed. Veronica Strong-Boag and Anita Fellman, 200-25. Toronto: Copp Clark Pitman, 1986.

Blackfoot Gallery Committee. *Nitsitapiisinni: The Story of the Blackfoot People.* Toronto: Key Porter Books, 2001.

Blackwood, Evelyn. *Female Desires: Same-Sex Relations and Transgender Practices across Cultures.* New York: Columbia University Press, 1999.

–. "Sexuality and Gender in Certain Native American Tribes: The Case of Cross-Gender Females." *Signs* 10, 11 (1984): 27-42.

Borst, Charlotte. *Catching Babies: The Professionalization of Childbirth, 1870-1920.* Cambridge, MA: Harvard University Press, 1995.

–. "Teaching Obstetrics at Home: Medical Schools and Home Delivery Services in the First Half of the Twentieth Century." *Bulletin of the History of Medicine* 72, 2 (1998): 220-45.

Bourgeault, Ivy Lynn. *Push! The Struggle for Midwifery in Ontario.* Montreal/Kingston: McGill-Queen's University Press, 2006.

Briggs, Charles, and Richard Bauman, "The Foundation of All Future Researches: Franz Boas, George Hunt, Native American Tests, and the Construction of Modernity." *American Quarterly* 51, 3 (1999): 479-528.

Brouwer, Ruth Compton. *New Women for God: Canadian Presbyterian Women and India Missions, 1876-1914.* Toronto: University of Toronto Press, 1990.

–. "Opening Doors through Social Service: Aspects of Women's Work in the Canadian Presbyterian Mission in Central India, 1871-1914." In *Prophets, Priests, and Prodigals: Readings in Canadian Religious History, 1608 to the Present,* ed. Mark McGowan and David Marshall, 241-61. Toronto: McGraw-Hill Ryerson, 1992.

Brown, Annora. *Old Man's Garden.* Toronto: Dent, 1954.

Brown, Jennifer. "A Cree Nurse in a Cradle of Methodism: Little Mary and the Egerton R. Young Family at Norway House and Berens River." In *Canadian Family History: Selected Readings,* ed. Bettina Bradbury, 90-110. Toronto: Copp Clark Pitman.

–. *Strangers in Blood: Fur Trade Company Families in Indian Country.* Vancouver: UBC Press, 1980.

Burnett, Kristin. "Aboriginal and White Women in the Publications of John Maclean, Egerton Ryerson Young, and John McDougall." In *Unsettled Pasts: Reconceiving the West through Women's History,* ed. Sarah Carter, Lesley Erickson, Patricia Roome, and Char Smith, 101-22. Calgary: University of Calgary Press, 2005.

Burton, Antoinette. *Burdens of History: British Feminists, Indian Women, and Imperial Culture, 1865-1915*. London: University of North Carolina Press, 1994.
—. "Contesting the Zenana: The Mission to Make Lady Doctors for India, 1874-1885." *Journal of British Studies* 35, 3 (1996): 368-97.
Carroll, Dena, and Cecilia Benoit. "Aboriginal Midwifery in Canada: Merging Traditional Practices and Modern Science." In *Reconceiving Midwifery*, ed. Ivy Bourgeault, Cecilia Benoit, and Robbi Davis-Floyd, 263-86. Montreal/Kingston: McGill-Queen's University Press, 2004.
Carter, Sarah. *Aboriginal People and Colonizers of Western Canada to 1900*. Toronto: University of Toronto Press, 1999.
—. *Capturing Women: The Manipulation of Cultural Imagery in Canada's Prairie West*. Montreal/Kingston: McGill-Queen's University Press, 1997.
—. "Categories and Terrains of Exclusion: Constructing the 'Indian Woman' in the Early Settlement Era in Western Canada." *Great Plains Quarterly* 13 (Summer 1993): 147-61.
—. "First Nations Women and Colonization on the Canadian Prairies, 1870s-1920s." In *Rethinking Canada: The Promise of Women's History*, ed. Veronica Strong-Boag, Mona Gleason, and Adele Perry, 135-48. 4th ed. Don Mills, ON: Oxford University Press, 2002.
—. *The Importance of Being Monogamous: Marriage and Nation Building in Western Canada to 1915*. Edmonton: Athabasca University Press/University of Alberta Press, 2008.
—. *Lost Harvests: Prairie Indian Reserve Farmers and Government Policy*. Montreal/Kingston: McGill-Queen's University Press, 1990.
Cashman, Tony. *Heritage of Service: The History of Nursing in Alberta*. Edmonton: Alberta Association of Registered Nurses, 1966.
Choquette, Robert. *The Oblate Assault on Canada's Northwest*. Ottawa: University of Ottawa Press, 1995.
Churchill, Elizabeth. "Tsuu T'ina: A History of a First Nations Community, 1890-1940." PhD diss., University of Calgary, 2000.
Cochrane and Area Historical Society, eds. *Big Hill Country: Cochrane and Area*. Cochrane, AB: Cochrane and Area Historical Society, 1977.
Colley, Kate Brighty. *While Rivers Flow: Stories of Early Alberta*. Saskatoon: Western Producer, 1970.
Comacchio, Cynthia. *"Nations Are Built of Babies": Saving Ontario's Mothers and Children, 1900-1940*. Montreal/Kingston: McGill Queen's University Press, 1993.
Comaroff, Jean. *Body of Power, Spirit of Resistance: The Culture and History of a South African People*. Chicago: University of Chicago Press, 1985.
Comaroff, Jean, and John Comaroff, eds. *Civil Society and the Political Imagination in Africa: Critical Perspectives*. Chicago: University of Chicago Press, 1999.
—. "Homemade Hegemony: Modernity, Domesticity, and Colonialism in South Africa." In *African Encounters with Domesticity*, ed. Karen Tranberg Hansen, 37-74. New Jersey: Rutgers, 1992.
Crowshoe, Reg, and Sybille Manneschmidt. *Akak'stiman: A Blackfoot Framework for Decision-Making and Mediation Processes*. Calgary: University of Calgary Press, 2001.
Cruickshank, Julie, Angela Sidney, Kitty Smith, and Annie Ned. *Life Lived Like a Story: Life Stories of Three Yukon Elders*. Lincoln/Vancouver: University of Nebraska Press/UBC Press, 1990.

Danylewycz, Marta. *Taking the Veil: An Alternative to Marriage, Motherhood, and Spinsterhood in Quebec, 1840-1920.* Toronto: McClelland and Stewart, 1987.

Darnell, Regna. *Invisible Genealogies: A History of Americanist Anthropology.* Lincoln: University of Nebraska Press, 2001.

Daviss, Betty-Anne. "Heeding Warnings from the Canary, the Whale and the Inuit: A Framework for Analyzing Competing Types of Knowledge about Childbirth." In *Childbirth and Authoritative Knowledge: Cross-Cultural Perspectives,* ed. Robbie Davis-Floyd and Carolyn Sargent, 441-73. Berkeley: University of California Press, 1997.

Decker, Jody. "Country Distempers: Deciphering Disease and Illness in Rupert's Land before 1870." In *Reading beyond Words: Contexts for Native History,* ed. Jennifer Brown and Elizabeth Vibert, 156-81. Peterborough, ON: Broadview Press, 1998.

–. "Tracing Historical Diffusion Patterns: The Case of the 1780-82 Smallpox Epidemic among the Indians of Western Canada." *Native Studies Review* 4, 1-2 (1988): 1-24.

Dempsey, Hugh. "The Blackfoot Indians." In *Native Peoples: The Canadian Experience,* ed. R. Bruce Morrison and C. Roderick Wilson, 381-413. 2nd ed. Toronto: McClelland and Stewart, 1995.

–. *Indian Tribes of Alberta.* Calgary: Glenbow-Alberta Institute, 1988.

–. "One Hundred Years of Treaty Seven." In *One Century Later: Western Canadian Reserve Indians since Treaty 7,* ed. Ian Getty and Donald Smith, 20-30. Vancouver: UBC Press, 1978.

Dobak, William. "Killing the Canadian Buffalo, 1821-1881." *Western Historical Quarterly* 27 (Spring 1996): 33-52.

Dodd, Dianne. "Advice to Parents: The Blue Books, Helen MacMurchy, MD, and the Federal Department of Health, 1920-34." *Canadian Bulletin of Medical History/Bulletin canadien d'histoire de la médecine* 8, 1 (1991): 203-30.

–. "Helen MacMurchy: Popular Midwifery and Maternity Services for Canadian Pioneer Women." In *Caring and Curing: Historical Perspectives on Women and Healing in Canada,* ed. Dianne Dodd and Deborah Gorham, 135-61. Ottawa: University of Ottawa Press, 1994.

Duffin, Jacalyn. *Langstaff: A Nineteenth-Century Medical Life.* Toronto: University of Toronto Press, 1993.

Emmerich, Lisa. "To Respect and Love and Seek the Ways of White Women: Field Matrons, the Office of Indian Affairs, and Civilization Policy, 1890-1938." PhD diss., University of Maryland, 1984.

Erickson, Paul, and Liam Murphy. *A History of Anthropological Theory.* 2nd ed. Peterborough, ON: Broadview Press, 2003.

Ettinger, Laura. "Mission to Mothers: Nuns, Latino Families, and the Founding of Santa Fe's Catholic Maternity Institute." In *Women, Health, and Nation: Canada and the United States since 1945,* ed. Georgina Feldberg, Molly Ladd Taylor, Allison Li, and Kathryn McPherson, 144-60. Montreal/Kingston: McGill-Queen's University Press, 2003.

Evans, Simon. *The Bar U: Canadian Ranching History.* Calgary: University of Calgary Press, 2004.

Ewers, John. *The Blackfeet: Raiders on the Northwestern Plains.* Norman: University of Oklahoma Press, 1958.

–. "Contraceptive Charms among the Plains Indians." *Plains Anthropologist* 15 (1970): 216-18.

–. *The Horse in Blackfeet Indian Culture: With Comparative Material from Other Western Tribes*. Washington, DC: Smithsonian Institution Press, 1955.
Feldberg, Georgina. *Disease and Class: Tuberculosis and the Shaping of Modern North American Society*. New Brunswick, NJ: Rutgers University Press, 1995.
Feldberg, Georgina, Molly Ladd Taylor, Allison Li, and Kathryn McPherson, eds. *Women, Health, and Nation: Canada and the United States since 1945*. Montreal/Kingston: McGill-Queen's University Press, 2003.
Flannery, Regina. *Ellen Smallboy: Glimpses of a Cree Woman's Life*. Montreal/Kingston: McGill-Queen's University Press, 1995.
Flint, Karen. "Competition, Race, and Professionalization: African Healers and White Medical Practitioners in Natal, South Africa, in the Early Twentieth Century." *Social History of Medicine* 14, 2 (2001): 199-221.
Flores, Dan. "Bison Ecology and Bison Diplomacy: The Southern Plains from 1800 to 1850." *Journal of American History* 78, 2 (1991): 465-85.
Francis, Daniel. *The Imaginary Indian: The Image of the Indian in Canadian Culture*. Vancouver: Arsenal Pulp Press, 1992.
Friesen, Gerald. *The Canadian Prairies: A History*. Toronto: University of Toronto Press, 1987.
Gagan, David, and Rosemary Gagan. *For Patients of Moderate Means: A Social History of the Voluntary Public General Hospital in Canada, 1890-1950*. Montreal/Kingston: McGill-Queen's University Press, 2002.
Gagan, Rosemary. "Gender, Work, and Zeal: Women Missionaries in Canada and Abroad." *Labour/Le Travail* 53 (2004): 1-18.
–. *A Sensitive Independence: Canadian Methodist Women Missionaries in Canada and the Orient, 1881-1925*. Montreal/Kingston: McGill-Queen's University Press, 1992.
Gerson, Carole. "Nobler Savages: Representations of Native Women in the Writings of Susanna Moodie and Catharine Parr Traill." *Journal of Canadian Studies* 32, 2 (1997-98): 5-21.
Gordon, Linda. "Internal Colonialism and Gender." In *Haunted by Empire: Geographies of Intimacy in North American History*, ed. Ann Laura Stoler, 427-68. Durham, NC: Duke University Press, 2006.
Graham-Cumming, G. "The Health of the Original Canadians, 1867-1967." *Medical Services Journal* 23, 2 (1967): 115-66.
Grant, John Webster. *Moon of Wintertime: Missionaries and the Indians of Canada in Encounter since 1534*. Toronto: University of Toronto Press, 1984.
Grant, Julia. *Raising Baby by the Book: The Education of American Mothers*. London: Yale University Press, 1998.
Hall, Catherine. "Commentary." In *Haunted by Empire: Geographies of Intimacy in North American History*, ed. Ann Laura Stoler, 452-68. Durham, NC: Duke University, 2006.
Halladay, Laurel. "We'll See You Next Year: Maternity Homes in Southern Saskatchewan in the First Half of the Twentieth Century." Master's thesis, Carleton University, 1996.
Halpern, Monda. *And on That Farm He Had a Wife: Ontario Farm Women and Feminism, 1900-1970*. Montreal/Kingston: McGill-Queen's University Press, 2001.
Hancock, Christin. "Sovereign Bodies: Women, Health Care, and Federal Indian Policy, 1890-1986." PhD diss., Brown University, 2006.
Handy-Marchello, Barbara. *Women of the Northern Plains: Gender and Settlement on the Homestead Frontier, 1870-1930*. Minneapolis: Minnesota Historical Society Press, 2005.

Hellson, John, and Morgan Gadd. *Ethnobotany of the Blackfoot Indians*. Ottawa: National Museums of Canada, 1974.

Higham, C.L. "A Hewer of Wood and Drover of Water": Expectations of Protestant Missionary Women on the Western Frontiers of Canada and the United States, 1830-1900." *Canadian Review of American Studies* 31, 1 (2001): 447-70.

—. *Noble, Wretched, and Redeemable: Protestant Missionaries to the Indians in Canada and the United States, 1820-1900*. Albuquerque: University of New Mexico Press, 2000.

—. "Saviours and Scientists: North American Protestant Missionaries and the Development of Anthropology." *Pacific Historical Review* 72, 4 (2003): 531-59.

Hine, Darlene Clark. *Black Women in White: Racial Conflict and Cooperation in the Nursing Profession, 1890-1950*. Bloomington: Indiana University Press, 1989.

Hume, Stephen. *Lilies and Fireweed: Frontier Women of British Columbia*. Madeira Park, BC: Harbour Publishing, 2004.

Hungry Wolf, Adolf. *The Blackfoot Papers – Volume One: Pikunni History and Culture*. Skookumchuck, BC: Good Medicine Cultural Foundation, 2006.

Hungry Wolf, Beverly. *The Ways of My Grandmothers*. New York: William Morrow and Company, 1980.

Indian and Northern Affairs Canada. Communications Branch. "Words First: An Evolving Terminology Relating to Aboriginal Peoples in Canada." Collections Canada. October 2002. http://www.collectionscanada.gc.ca/webarchives/20071115071229/http://www.ainc-inac.gc.ca/pr/pub/wf/pdf_e.html.

Isenberg, Andrew. *The Destruction of the Buffalo*. Cambridge: Cambridge University Press, 2000.

Jacobs, Margaret. *Endgendered Encounters: Feminism and Pueblo Culture, 1879-1934*. Lincoln: University of Nebraska Press, 1999.

—. "The Great White Mother: Maternalism and American Indian Child Removal in the American West." In *One Step Over the Line: Toward a History of Women in the North American Wests,* ed. Elizabeth Jameson and Sheila McManus, 191-214. Edmonton: Athabasca University Press/University of Alberta Press, 2008.

—. "Working on the Domestic Frontier: American Indian Domestic Servants in White Women's Household in the San Francisco Area, 1920-1940," *Frontiers* 28, 1-2 (2007): 165-99.

Jamieson, Kathryn. *Indian Women and the Law in Canada: Citizens Minus*. Ottawa: Advisory Council on the Status of Women, 1978.

Janes, Sharyn. "Transcultural Nursing and Global Health." In *Essentials of Community-Based Nursing,* ed. Karen Saucier Lundy and Sharyn Janes, 122-37. Sudbury, ON: Jones and Bartlett, 2003.

Janiewski, Dolores. "Gendered Colonialism: The Woman Question in Settler Society." In *Nation, Empire, Colony: Historicizing Gender and Race,* eds. Ruth Roach Pierson, Nupur Chaudhuri, and Beth McAuley, 57-76. Bloomington: Indian University Press, 1998.

Jasen, Patricia. "Race, Culture, and the Colonization of Childbirth in Northern Canada." *Social History of Medicine* 10, 3 (1997): 383-400.

Jensen, Joan. *Calling This Place Home: Women on the Wisconsin Frontier, 1850-1925*. Minneapolis: Minnesota Historical Society Press, 2006.

Johnston, Alex. *Plants and the Blackfoot*. Lethbridge: Historical Society of Alberta, 1987.

Jones, David. *Empire of Dust: Settling and Abandoning the Prairie Dry Belt*. Edmonton: University of Alberta Press, 1987.

Kehoe, Alice. "How the Ancient Peigans Lived." *Research in Economic Anthropology* 14 (1993): 87-105.

—. Introduction to *Mythology of the Blackfoot Indians,* by Clark Wissler and D.C. Duvall, v-xxxiii. Lincoln: University of Nebraska Press, 1995.

Kelcy, Barbara. *Alone in Silence: European Women in the Canadian North before 1940.* Montreal/Kingston: McGill-Queen's University Press, 2001.

Kelm, Mary-Ellen. *Colonizing Bodies: Aboriginal Health and Healing in British Columbia, 1900-1950.* Vancouver: UBC Press, 1998.

—. "Diagnosing the Discursive Indian: Medicine, Gender, and the Dying Race," *Ethnohistory* 52, 2 (2005): 371-406.

—. "A Scandalous Procession: Residential Schooling and Re/formation of Aboriginal Bodies, 1900-1950." *Native Studies Review* 11, 2 (1996): 51-88.

Kelton, Paul. "Avoiding the Smallpox Spirits: Colonial Epidemics and Southeastern Indian Survival." *Ethnohistory* 51, 1 (2004): 45-71.

Kennedy, Dan. *Recollections of an Assiniboine Chief.* Edited by James Stevens. Toronto: McClelland and Stewart, 1972.

Kipp, Darrell Robes. Introduction to *Blackfeet Tales of Glacier National Park,* by James Shultz, vi-ix. Helena, MO: Riverbend Publishing, 2002 [1917].

Klein, Alan. "The Political-Economy of Gender: A Nineteenth-Century Plains Indian Case Study." In *The Hidden Half: Studies of Plains Indian Women,* ed. Patricia Albers and Beatrice Medicine, 143-73. Lanham, MD: University Press of America, 1983.

Kozak, Nadine. "Advice and Rural Prairie Realities: National and Prairie Scientific Motherhood Advice, 1920-29." In *Unsettled Pasts: Reconceiving the West through Women's History,* ed. Sarah Carter, Lesley Erickson, Patricia Roome, and Char Smith, 179-204. Calgary: University of Calgary Press, 2005.

Langford, Nanci. "Childbirth on the Canadian Prairies, 1880-1939." In *Telling Tales: Essays in Western Women's History,* ed. Catherine Cavanaugh and Randi Warne, 147-73. Vancouver: UBC Press, 2000.

Leavitt, Judith, and Ronald Numbers. "Sickness and Health in America: An Overview." In *Sickness and Health in America,* ed. Judith Leavitt and Ronald Numbers, 3-10. Madison: University of Wisconsin Press, 1997.

Leighton, Douglas. "A Victorian Civil Servant at Work: Lawrence Vankoughnet and the Canadian Indian Department, 1874-1893." In *As Long as the Sun Shines and Water Flows: A Reader in Canadian Native Studies,* ed. Ian Getty and Antoine Lussier, 104-19. Vancouver: UBC Press, 1983.

Levine, Philippa. *Prostitution, Race, and Politics: Policing Venereal Disease in the British Empire.* New York: Routledge, 2003.

Lewis, Oscar. "Manly-Hearted Women among the North Peigan." *American Anthropologist,* n.s., 43, 2 (1941): 173-87.

Lutz, John. "Gender and Work in Lekwammen Families, 1843-1970." In *Gendered Pasts: Historical Essays in Femininity and Masculinity in Canada,* ed. Kathryn McPherson, Cecilia Morgan, and Nancy Forestell, 80-105. Don Mills, ON: Oxford University Press, 1999.

—. "Relating to the Country: The Lekwammen and the Extension of European Settlement." In *Beyond the City Limits: Rural History in British Columbia,* ed. R.W. Sandwell, 17-32. Vancouver: UBC Press, 1999.

Lux, Maureen. *Medicine That Walks: Disease, Medicine, and Canadian Plains Native People, 1880-1940*. Toronto: University of Toronto Press, 2001.

–. "Perfect Subjects: Race, Tuberculosis, and the Qu'Appelle BCG Vaccine Trial." *Canadian Bulletin of Medical History/Bulletin canadien d'histoire de la médecine* 15 (1998): 277-95.

MacDonald, Margaret. *Work in the Field of Birth: Midwifery Narratives of Nature, Tradition, and Home*. Nashville, TN: Vanderbilt University Press, 2007.

MacEwan, Grant. *... And Mighty Women Too: Stories of Notable Western Canadian Women*. Saskatoon: Western Producer Books, 1975.

Martin, John Julius. *The Prairie Hub: An Outline of Early Western Events from the Hand Hills to the Buffalo Hills*. Rosebud, AB: Strathmore Standard, 1967.

McCallum, M.G. "The Alberta Department of Public Health." In *The Federal and Provincial Health Services in Canada*, ed. R.D. Defries, 109-22. 2nd ed. Ottawa: Canadian Public Health Association, 1962.

McClintock, Anne. *Imperial Leather: Race, Gender, and Sexuality in the Colonial Contest*. New York: Routledge, 1995.

–. "No Longer in a Future Heaven: Gender, Race, and Nationalism." In *Dangerous Liaisons: Gender, Nation, and Postcolonial Perspectives*, ed. Anne McClintock, Amir Rashid Mufti, and Ella Shohat, 89-113. Minneapolis: University of Minnesota Press, 1997.

McCrady, David. *Living with Strangers: The Nineteenth-Century Sioux and the Canadian-American Borderlands*. Lincoln: University of Nebraska Press, 2006.

McDowell, Linda. *Gender, Identity, and Place: Understanding Feminist Geographies*. Minneapolis: University of Minnesota Press, 1999.

McIntyre, Michael Lee. "Sarcee Demography." Master's thesis, University of Calgary, 1975.

McLaren, Angus. "Keep Your Seats and Face Facts: Western Canadian Women's Discussion of Birth Control in the 1920s," *Canadian Bulletin of Medical History/Bulletin canadien d'histoire de la médecine* 8, 2 (1991): 189-201.

–. *Reproductive Rituals: The Perception of Fertility in England from the Sixteenth to the Nineteenth Century*. London: Methuen and Co., 1984.

McManus, Sheila. *The Line Which Separates: Race, Gender, and the Making of the Alberta-Montana Borderlands*. Lincoln: University of Nebraska Press, 2005.

McMillan, Alan. *Native Peoples and Cultures of Canada: An Anthropological Overview*. Vancouver: Douglas and McIntyre, 1995.

McPherson, Kathryn. *Bedside Matters: The Transformation of Canadian Nursing, 1900-1990*. Toronto: Oxford University Press, 1996.

–. "Nursing and Colonization: The Work of Indian Health Service Nurses in Manitoba." In *Women, Health, and Nation: Canada and the United States since 1945*, ed. Georgina Feldberg, Molly Ladd Taylor, Allison Li, and Kathryn McPherson, 223-46. Montreal/Kingston: McGill-Queen's University Press, 2003.

Medicine, Beatrice. "Warrior Women: Sex Role Alternatives for Plains Indian Women." In *The Hidden Half: Studies of Plains Indian Women*, ed. Patricia Albers and Beatrice Medicine, 267-80. Lanham, MD: University Press of America, 1983.

Meijer Drees, Laurie. "Reserve Hospitals and Medical Officers: Health Care and Indian Peoples in Southern Alberta, 1890s-1930s." *Prairie Forum* 21, 2 (1996): 149-76.

–. "Reserve Hospitals in Southern Alberta, 1890-1930." *Native Studies Review* 9, 1 (1993-94): 93-110.

Meijer Drees, Laurie, and Lesley McBain. "Nursing and Native Peoples in Northern Saskatchewan, 1930-1950s." *Canadian Bulletin of Medical History/Bulletin canadien d'histoire de la médecine* 18 (2001): 43-65.

Meili, Dianne. *Those Who Know: Profiles of Alberta's Native Elders*. Edmonton: NeWest Press, 1991.

Melainey, Mary, and Barbara Sherriff. "Adjusting Our Perceptions: Historical and Archaeological Evidence of Winter on the Plains of Western Canada." *Plains Anthropologist* 1, 158 (1996): 333-57.

Melchior, Florence. "Nursing Student Labour, Education, and Patient Care at the Medicine Hat General Hospital, Alberta, 1890-1930." PhD diss., University of Calgary, 2004.

Milloy, John. *A National Crime: The Canadian Government and the Residential School System, 1879 to 1986*. Winnipeg: University of Manitoba Press, 1999.

Mitchinson, Wendy. *Giving Birth in Canada, 1900-1950*. Toronto: University of Toronto Press, 2002.

Mohatt, Gerald, and Joseph Eagle Elk. *The Price of a Gift: A Lakota Healer's Story*. Lincoln: University of Nebraska Press, 2000.

Mountain Horse, Mike. *My People the Bloods*. Calgary: Glenbow-Alberta Institute, 1979.

Muir, Elizabeth Gillian, and Marilyn Fardig Whiteley. "Introduction: Putting Together the Puzzle of Canadian Women's Christian Work." In *Changing Roles of Women within the Christian Church in Canada*, ed. Elizabeth Gillian Muir and Marilyn Fardig Whiteley, 3-16. Toronto: University of Toronto Press, 1995.

Nestel, Sheryl. *Obstructed Labour: Race and Gender in the Re-emergence of Midwifery*. Vancouver: UBC Press, 2006.

Newell, Dianne. "Belonging – Out of Place: Women's Travelling Stories from the Western Edge." In *Contact Zones: Aboriginal and Settler Women in Canada's Colonial Past*, ed. Katie Pickles and Myra Rutherdale, 246-71. Vancouver: UBC Press, 2005.

O'Neil, John, and Patricia Kaufert. "Irniktakpunga! Sex Determination and the Inuit Struggle for Birthing Rights in Northern Canada." In *Conceiving the New World Order: The Global Politics of Reproduction*, 59-73. Berkeley: University of California Press, 1995.

Pagh, Nancy. *At Home Afloat: Women on the Waters of the Pacific Northwest*. Calgary: University of Calgary Press, 2001.

Palmer, Howard, and Tamara Palmer. *Alberta: A New History*. Edmonton: Hurtig Publishers, 1990.

Parascandola, John. "The Introduction of Antibiotics into Therapeutics." In *Sickness and Health in America: Readings in the History of Medicine and Public Health*, ed. Judith Leavitt and Ronald Numbers, 102-12. Madison: University of Wisconsin Press, 1997.

Paul, Pauline. "The Contribution of the Grey Nuns to the Development of Nursing in Canada: Historiographical Issues." *Canadian Bulletin of Medical History/Bulletin canadien d'histoire de la médecine* 11 (1994): 207-17.

–. "A History of the Edmonton General Hospital, 1895-1970: 'Be Faithful to the Duties of Your Calling.'" PhD diss., University of Alberta, 1994.

Peacock, Sandra Leslie. "Piikani Ethnobotany: Traditional Plant Knowledge of the Piikani Peoples of the Northwestern Plains." Master's thesis, University of Calgary, 1992.

Perry, Adele. "From the Hot-Bed of Vice to the Good and Well-Ordered Christian Home: First Nations' Housing and Reform in Nineteenth-Century British Columbia." *Ethnohistory* 50, 4 (2003): 587-610.

–. *On the Edge of Empire: Gender, Race, and the Making of British Columbia, 1849-1871.* Toronto: University of Toronto Press, 2001.
Peterson, Lester. *The Story of the Sechelt Nation.* Sechelt, BC: Sechelt Indian Band, 1990.
Pettipas, Katherine. *Severing the Ties That Bind: Government Repression of Indigenous Religious Ceremonies on the Prairies.* Winnipeg: University of Manitoba Press, 1994.
Pickles, Katie, and Myra Rutherdale. "Introduction." In *Contact Zones: Aboriginal and Settler Women in Canada's Colonial Past,* ed. Katie Pickles and Myra Rutherdale, 1-14. Vancouver: UBC Press, 2005.
Porter, Andrew. *Religion vs. Empire: British Protestant Missions and Overseas Expansions, 1700-1914.* Manchester: Manchester University Press, 2004.
Pratt, Mary Louise. *Imperial Eyes: Travel Writing and Transculturation.* London: Routledge, 1992.
Rafael, Vincente L. "Colonial Domesticity: Engendering Race at the Edge of Empire, 1899-1920." In *White Love and Other Events in Filipino History,* ed. Vincente Rafael, 52-75. Durham, NC: Duke University Press, 2007.
–. *Colonial Domesticity: White Women and US Rule in the Philippines.* Durham, NC: Duke University Press, 1995.
Regular, W. Keith. *Neighbour and Networks: The Blood Tribe and the Southern Alberta Economy, 1884-1939.* Calgary: University of Calgary Press, 2009.
Reifel, Nancy. "American Indian Views of Public Health Nursing, 1930-1950." *American Indian Culture and Research Journal* 23, 3 (1999): 143-54.
Richardson, Sharon. "Alberta's Provincial Travelling Clinic, 1924-42." *Canadian Bulletin of Medical History/Bulletin canadien d'histoire* 19 (2002): 245-63.
–. "Frontier Health Care: Alberta's District and Municipal Nursing Services, 1919 to 1976." *Alberta History* 46, 1 (1998): 2-9.
Roe, Frank Gilbert. *The Indian and the Horse.* Norman: University of Oklahoma Press, 1955.
Rogers, Naomi. *Dirt and Disease: Polio before FDR.* New Brunswick, NJ: Rutgers University Press, 1992.
Roome, Patricia. "From One Whose Home Is among the Indians: Henrietta Muir Edwards and Aboriginal Peoples." In *Unsettled Pasts: Reconceiving the West through Women's History,* ed. Sarah Carter, Lesley Erickson, Patricia Roome, and Char Smith, 47-78. Calgary: University of Calgary Press, 2005.
Ross-Kerr, Janet. *Prepared to Care: Nurses and Nursing in Alberta.* Edmonton: University of Alberta Press, 1998.
Ruffing-Rahal, Mary Ann. "The Navajo Experience of Elizabeth Forster, Public Health Nurse." *Nursing History Review* 3 (1995): 173-88.
Rutherdale, Myra. "Revisiting Colonization through Gender: Anglican Missionary Women in the Pacific Northwest and the Arctic, 1860-1945." *BC Studies,* no. 104 (Winter 1994): 3-23.
–. "She Was a Ragged Little Thing: Missionaries, Embodiment, and Refashioning Aboriginal Womanhood in Northern Canada." In *Contact Zones: Aboriginal and Settler Women in Canada's Colonial Past,* ed. Katie Pickles and Myra Rutherdale, 228-45. Vancouver: UBC Press, 2005.
–. *Women and the White Man's God: Gender and Race in the Canadian Mission Field.* Vancouver: UBC Press, 2002.
Samek, Hana. *The Blackfoot Confederacy, 1880-1920: A Comparative Study of Canada and United States Indian Policy.* Albuquerque: University of New Mexico Press, 1987.

Sandelowski, Margarete. *Devices and Desires: Gender, Technology, and American Nursing.* Chapel Hill, ND: University of North Carolina Press, 2000.

Sangster, Joan. *Regulating Girls and Women: Sexuality, Family, and the Law in Ontario, 1920-1960.* Toronto: Oxford University Press, 2001.

Scott-Brown, Joan. "Stoney Ethnobotany: An Indication of Cultural Change amongst Stoney Women of Morley Alberta." Master's thesis, University of Calgary, 1977.

Secoy, Frank Raymond. *Changing Military Patterns of the Great Plains.* New York: J.J. Augustin, 1953.

Service, Elman. *The Hunters.* New Jersey: Prentice-Hall, 1966.

–. *Primitive Social Organization: An Evolutionary Perspective.* New York: Random House, 1962.

–. *Profiles in Ethnology.* 3rd ed. New York: Harper and Row, 1978.

Shah, Nayan. "Cleansing Motherhood: Hygiene and the Culture of Domesticity in San Francisco's Chinatown, 1875-1900." In *Gender, Sexuality, and Colonial Modernities,* ed. Antoinette Burton, 19-34. London: Routledge, 1999.

Shewell, Hugh. *Enough to Keep Them Alive: Indian Welfare in Canada, 1873 to 1965.* Toronto: University of Toronto Press, 2004.

Shimkin, Demitri. "The Introduction of the Horse." In *Handbook of North American Indians,* Vol. 11, ed. Warren D'Azevedo, 517-24. Washington, DC: Smithsonian Institution Press, 1986.

Silverman, Eliane Leslau. *The Last Best West: Women on the Alberta Frontier, 1880-1930.* Calgary: Fifth House, 1998.

Smith, Andrea. *Conquest: Sexual Violence and American Indian Genocide.* Cambridge: SouthEnd Press, 2005.

Smith, Sherry. *Reimagining Indians: Native Americans through Anglo Eyes, 1880-1940.* New York: Oxford University Press, 2000.

Smith, Susan. *Japanese American Midwives: Culture, Community, and Health Politics, 1880-1950.* Urbana: University of Illinois Press, 2005.

–. "White Nurses, Black Midwives, and Public Health in Mississippi, 1920-1950." *Nursing History Review* 2 (1994): 29-49.

Smith-Rosenberg, Carroll. "Captured Subjects/Savage Others: Violently Engendering the New American." *Gender and History* 5, 2 (1993): 177-95.

Smith, Sherry. *Reimagining Indians: Native Americans through Anglo Eyes, 1880-1940.* New York: Oxford University Press, 2000.

Smits, David. "The Frontier Army and the Destruction of the Buffalo, 1865-1883." In *Uncommon Ground: Rethinking the Human Place in Nature,* ed. William Cronon, 171-85. New York: W.W. Norton, 1995.

Sproule-Jones, Megan. "Crusading for the Forgotten: Dr. Peter Bryce, Public Health, and Prairie Native Residential Schools." *Canadian Bulletin of Medical History/Bulletin canadien d'histoire* 13, 2 (1996): 199-224.

Spry, Irene. *The Palliser Expedition: An Account of John Palliser's British North American Expedition, 1857-1860.* Toronto: Macmillan, 1963.

Stewart, Irene, ed. *These Were Our Yesterdays: A History of District Nursing in Alberta.* Calgary: Friesen Printers, 1979.

Stocking, George Jr. *The Ethnographers' Magic and Other Essays in the History of Anthropology.* Madison: University of Wisconsin Press, 1992.

Stoler, Ann Laura. *Carnal Knowledge and Imperial Power: Race and the Intimate in Colonial Rule*. Berkeley: University of California Press, 2002.

–. "Tense and Tender Ties: The Politics of Comparison in North American History and (Post) Colonial Studies." In *Haunted by Empire: Geographies of Intimacy in North American History*, ed. Ann Laura Stoler, 23-67. Durham, NC: Duke University Press, 2006.

Strong-Boag, Veronica, and Kathryn McPherson. "The Confinement of Women: Childbirth and Hospitalization in Vancouver, 1919-1939." *BC Studies*, nos. 69 and 70 (Spring-Summer 1986): 142-74.

Sundstrom, Linea. "Smallpox Used Them Up: References to Epidemic Disease in Northern Plains Winter Counts, 1714-1920." *Ethnohistory* 44, 2 (1997): 305-29.

Sutherland, Neil. *Children in English-Canadian Society: Framing the Twentieth-Century Consensus*. Waterloo: Wilfred Laurier University Press, 1978 [2000].

Taylor, Colin, and Hugh Dempsey. *With Eagle Tail: Arnold Lupson and Thirty Years among the Sarcee, Blackfoot, and Stoney Indians on the North American Plains*. New York: Salamander, 1999.

Taylor, William. Foreword to *The Indians of Canada*, by Diamond Jenness. v-x. Toronto: University of Toronto Press, 1977.

Thompson, Judy. *Recording Their Story: James and the Tahltan*. Vancouver: Douglas and McIntyre, 2007.

Thomson, Gerald. "A Baby Show Means Work in the Hardest Sense: The Better Baby Contests of the Vancouver and New Westminster Local Councils of Women, 1913-1929." *BC Studies*, no. 128 (Winter 2000-01): 5-36.

Titley, E. Brian. *A Narrow Vision: Duncan Campbell Scott and the Administration of Indian Affairs in Canada*. Vancouver: UBC Press, 1986.

–. *The Indian Commissioners: Agents of the State and Indian Policy in Canada's Prairie West, 1873-1932*. Edmonton: University of Alberta Press, 2009.

Tobias, John. "Protection, Civilization, Assimilation: An Outline History of Canada's Indian Policy." In *As Long as the Sun Shines and Water Flows: A Reader in Native Canadian Studies*, ed. Ian Getty and Antoine Lussier, 39-55. Vancouver: UBC Press, 1983.

Tomes, Nancy. "The Private Side of Public Health: Sanitary Science, Domestic Hygiene, and the Germ Theory, 1870-1900." In *Sickness and Health in America: Readings in the History of Medicine and Public Health,* ed. Judith Leavitt and Ronald Numbers, 506-28. Madison: University of Wisconsin Press, 1997.

Treaty 7 Elders and Tribal Council, with Walter Hildebrandt, Dorothy First Rider, and Sarah Carter. *The True Spirit and Original Intent of Treaty 7*. Montreal/Kingston: McGill-Queen's University Press, 1996.

Trigger, Bruce. "The French Presence in Huronia: The Structure of Franco-Huron Relations in the First Half of the 17th-Century." In *Readings in Canadian History: Pre-Confederation*, ed. Douglas Francis and Donald Smith, 21-47. 6th ed. Toronto: Nelson Thomas, 2002.

Valverde, Mariana. *The Age of Light, Soap, and Water: Moral Reform in English Canada, 1885-1925*. Toronto: McClelland and Stewart, 1991.

Van Kirk, Sylvia. *Many Tender Ties: Women in Fur-Trade Society, 1670-1870*. Winnipeg: Watson and Dwyer, 1980.

Vaughan, Megan. *Curing Their Ills: Colonial Power and African Illness*. Stanford, CA: Stanford University Press, 1991.

Vibert, Elizabeth. "Real Men Hunt Buffalo: Masculinity, Race, and Class in British Fur Traders' Narratives." In *Gender and History in Canada,* ed. Joy Parr and Mark Rosenfeld, 50-67. Mississauga, ON: Copp Clark, 1996.
–. *Traders' Tales: Narratives of Cultural Encounters in the Columbia Plateau, 1807-1946.* Norman: University of Oklahoma Press, 1997.
Waldram, James, D. Ann Herring, and T. Kue Young. *Aboriginal Health in Canada: Historical, Cultural, and Epidemiological Perspectives.* 1st ed. Toronto: University of Toronto Press, 1999.
White, Luise. *Speaking with Vampires: Rumour and History in East and Central Africa.* Berkeley: University of California Press, 2000.
White, Pamela Margaret. "Restructuring the Domestic Sphere: Prairie Indian Women on Reserves – Image, Ideology, and State Policy, 1880-1930." PhD diss., McGill University, 1987.
Wood, Patricia. "Pressured from All Sides: The February 1913 Surrender of the Northeast Corner of the Tsuu T'ina Nation." *Journal of Historical Geography* 30, 1 (2004): 113-30.
Woywitka, Anne. "Pioneers in Sickness and in Health." *Alberta History* 49, 1 (2001): 16-20.
Young, Judith. "'Monthly' Nurses, Sick Nurses, and Midwives in 19th-Century Toronto." *Canadian Bulletin of Medical History/Bulletin canadien d'histoire* 21, 2 (2004): 281-302.
–. "Recent Health Trends in the Native American Population." In *Changing Numbers, Changing Needs: American Indian Demography and Public Health,* eds. Gary Sandefur, Ronald Rindfuss, and Barney Cohen, 53-76. Washington, DC: National Academy Press, 1996.
Zaharia, Flora, and Leo Fox, eds. *Kitomahkitapiiminnooniksi: Stories from Our Elders.* Vols. 1-3. Edmonton: Donahue House, 1995.

Index

Abel, Emily, 114
abortion, 60, 154
Adam, François, 52
Adams, Annmarie, 146
adenitis, 136
agriculture, 28, 26-27, 48-49, 71
Albers, Patricia, 42
Alberta District Nursing Service, 143, 156
Alberta Railway and Coal Company, 82
Allison, John, 53
Allison, Susan, 53
American Fur Trade Company, 24
American Museum of Natural History, 38
Ames, Herbert, 31
Angel, Michael, 40
anthropology, 36-43, 167
Apsálooke (Crow), 24
Arrowtop, Mrs. Philip, 164-65
Arrowwood Creek, 26
arthritis, 53
assimilation, 36, 64, 69, 83, 119, 128, 167
Assiniboine, 18, 24, 55. *See also* Nakoda (Stoney)
Assiniboine River, 51

Bailey Price, Elizabeth, 63
band formation, 19-20
Banff National Park, 18, 82

Bare Shin Bone, Annie, 126
Barker, Sarah Ann, 71
Battleford District, 52, 55, 58, 65, 78
Bearspaw, Peter, 62
Beaver Creek, 27
Belly River, 26
Bennett, R.B., 134-35
Big Plume, 76
Biggs, Lesley, 57
Blackfoot. *See* Siksika (Blackfoot) *under* Blackfoot Nation
Blackfoot Hospital, 32, 92-93, 98, 102-4, 107, 110-11, 115-16, 129, 131, 137, 139, 159, 162
Blackfoot Lodge Tales (Grinnell), 38, 41
Blackfoot Nation: Kainai (Blood), 6, 10, 15, 17, 21-22, 25-38, 30, 39, 42, 71, 74, 76, 94, 118, 123-25, 131, 139, 141, 148, 150, 157, 170; Siksika (Blackfoot), 6, 10, 15, 17, 20–22, 25-28, 30, 73-76, 116-17, 136, 147, 159, 161, 163-66, 170; Piikani (Peigan), 6, 10, 15, 17, 21-22, 25, 27-30, 38, 41-42, 74, 80, 91, 110, 117, 131, 134, 170
Blackfoot Reserve, 37-39, 41, 58-59, 76, 95, 106, 109-10, 117, 132, 138, 146, 148, 150, 158

Blackwood, Evelyn, 24
Blood. *See* Kainai (Blood) *under* Blackfoot Nation
Blood Hospital, 32, 97, 99-104, 107, 109-11, 116, 118-19, 125, 129-31, 133, 137-40, 142, 151, 157, 159-60
Blood Reserve, 30, 58, 71, 74, 80-81, 85, 91, 94-95, 98, 103, 109-10, 112, 115, 117, 126, 132-33, 137, 139-41, 150
BNA Act, 31-32
Boas, Franz, 12, 38
Bompas, Charlotte Selina, 51
Bompas, William C., 51
Booth, Alma, 104
Bourne, Rev. H.T., 75
Bow River District, 27, 59
Bradley, Dr. Gerald, 56
Brandon, Annie, 149-50
Bray, Charles, 59
Brown, Jennifer, 64
Brown, Kate, 73, 75-76, 80
Bryce, Dr. Peter H., 95-97, 127, 133
buffalo hunt, 11, 18-23, 25, 35-36, 42-43, 59, 76, 169
Bull Horn School, 81

Calgary (AB), 10, 13, 26-27, 49, 55, 60, 65, 84, 94, 104, 109, 124, 130, 137, 142-43, 160
Calgary General Hospital, 82, 97
Canadian Arctic Expedition, 13
Canadian Pacific Railway (CPR), 28, 48, 82
Canadian Tuberculosis Association, 31, 96
Cardston (AB), 49, 129-31, 140-42
Carrier, Marion, 42
Carter, Sarah, 47, 78
Catholic Maternity Institute, 160
Cecil, Mary, 59-60, 63, 66
chicken pox, 137
Chief Coward, Mrs. Victor, 164-66
child care, 105-6, 127, 135-36, 144-48, 151-52, 154, 173, 175
Child Welfare Clinic, 143
childbirth, 8-10, 13, 15, 35-36, 43-45, 47-48, 50, 52-55, 53, 56-59, 65, 137, 146-47, 149, 152-63, 167, 170-75. *See also* midwifery; pregnancy
Christian Guardian, 74
Christian Missionary Society, 81, 108, 113
Church Missionary Society, 51, 73, 81
Church Women's Mission Aid Society (Toronto), 73
Clendennan, Dr. A.E., 143
coal, 49
Coalbanks Mine Hospital, 82
colonialism, 4-11, 14, 48, 64, 66, 78, 119, 173
Columbia University, 12
Comacchio, Cynthia, 105
Comaroff, Jean, 6
Comaroff, Jeff, 6
contraception, 13, 60, 153-55, 163-67
Cornish, F.C., 60, 63-64
Crane Bear, Tony, 125
Cree, 18, 24, 51, 55-57, 59, 64
Criminal Code, 65, 163
Crooked Lake (SK), 52
Crow. See Apsálooke (Crow), 24
Crowfoot Creek, 26
Crowshoe, Reg, 20

Dakota, 38
Dauphin (MB), 53
Daviss, Betty-Anne, 155
Decker, Jody, 25
Department of Indian Affairs (DIA), 6-10, 13, 15, 27, 29, 31-32, 48, 55, 64, 67, 73, 75, 79-80, 82-87, 89-96, 98, 100, 105-7, 109-13, 117-36, 138, 140-57, 159-60, 162-63, 168, 172-75
Department of Mines and Natural Resources, 130
Department of Public Health, 143
Department of the Interior, 96
Dewdney, Edgar, 85
Dilworth, W.J., 103, 117, 126
diphtheria, 132
Dominion Lands Act, 28
Dominion Survey, 59
Drees, Laurie Meijer, 100-1
Drumheller (AB), 143

Duvall, David C., 38, 43-44, 163, 166
dysentery, 59, 137

Eagle Tail Feathers, Frank, 162
economic geography, 10
Edmonton (AB), 49, 55, 112, 143
Edmonton General Hospital, 97
Edwards, Henrietta Muir, 131
Edwards, Dr. O.C., 111, 124, 131, 139, 159
Elbow River, 27
Elk Point, 56
Emmerich, Lisa, 128
Enough to Keep Them Alive (Shewell), 30
Erie (PA), 98
ethnobotany, 42, 45, 50, 52-54, 58-59, 78, 126, 162, 166-67, 170, 174-75
ethnography, 36-43, 167
Ettinger, Laura, 160
Ewers, John, 29
exorcism, 38

Farwell Bradley, Irene, 56
Faunt, Joseph Thomas, 150, 157
Favel, Thomas, 51
federal government, 4-7, 15, 26, 28, 30-32, 36, 68, 83, 85-86, 91-93, 110, 122, 127, 134, 141, 156, 167, 174
field matrons, 128-29, 144, 149, 151, 152, 158
First Rider, George, 166
First World War, 15, 49, 98, 115, 130-31, 139, 152, 156-57
Fish Creek, 27
Flint, Karen, 50
Forster, Elizabeth, 113-14
Fort Calgary, 27
Fort Chipewyan, 51
Fort Edmonton, 24, 58, 69, 82
Fort Macleod, 26-27, 65, 82, 84-85, 49, 124, 160
Fort Pelly, 51
Fort Simpson, 51
Frog Lake , 55
fur trade, 18, 24, 36, 47, 51, 52, 59, 78, 123

Gadd, Morgan, 166-67
Gagan, David, 157
Gagan, Rosemary, 157
gallstones, 126
gender, 4, 6-7, 22-23, 35-36, 42-43, 45, 50-51, 65, 69, 78, 100-1, 121, 135, 152, 167, 169-70, 174-75
General and Marine Hospital, 97
Girard, Dr. Francis Xavier, 85
Gleichen (AB), 78, 108
Glenbow Archives, 13-14, 63
Goldfrank, Esther, 160-62, 164, 166
Gooderham, George, 138, 146-47, 158-59
Gooderham, J.H., 98, 117
Goodstriker, Rufus, 39, 42, 125-26
Gordon, Linda, 5
Graham, Thomas, 126, 133, 147
Graham, William Morris, 126
Grant, John Webster, 70
Great Depression, 31, 49, 130
Greer, Annie, 53-54
Grey Nuns, 71-72, 81-82, 97-98, 103, 107, 119, 129-30, 139-41, 159. *See also* Sisters of Charity
Grinnell, George Bird, 29, 36-39, 41-42; *Blackfoot Lodge Tales,* 38, 41
grippe, 136
Guelph General Hospital, 108

Hanks, Lucien, 125, 159, 161
Haynes, W.R., 90-91
Hellson, John, 166-67
Herring, D. Ann, 100
High River (AB), 71, 109
Hill, Maud, 137, 148
Hoade, Elizabeth, 82
Holy Cross Hospital, 82, 160
Home Gun, Mrs. Pete, 166
Hôpital Notre-Dame, 98
Hopkins, Monica, 61-62
Horn Society, 20
horses, 24, 35
Hudson's Bay Company, 28, 48
Huncomb, Agnes, 136
Hungry Wolf, Beverly, 162, 165
Huron Women's Auxiliary, 94

Index

Hyde, W. Julius, 159
hygiene and sanitation, 96-97, 105, 122, 127-29, 138, 144, 148-49, 151, 173
hypnotism, 38

incantation, 38, 40
Indian Act, 29, 64-65, 127, 146
Indian Health Services (IHS), 4, 15, 32, 89, 91, 114, 127, 129, 130, 142-43, 172-73
infant mortality, 134-36, 144-46, 154, 156-57, 159, 173
influenza, 132
Ing, Marchmont, 104
Isenberg, Andrew, 24

James Bay, 56
Jameson, Ethel, 56
Jasen, Patricia, 155
Jenness, Diamond, 13, 161

Kainai (Blood). *See under* Blackfoot Nation
Kanazawa (Japan), 108
Kaufert, Patricia, 155
Kelcy, Barbara, 9
Kelm, Mary-Ellen, 7, 80, 110
Kennedy, Dr. Alan, 118, 137-39, 157
Kidd, John, 142

Lac Sainte-Anne, 82
Lacombe, Father Albert, 91-92
Lafferty, Dr. James, 55, 110, 124
Laing, Margaret, 79, 108-9
Lake of the Woods, 18
Lake Winnipeg, 18
Langford, Nanci, 65
Lawrence, Mary, 54-55
Le Drew (nurse), 132-33
Legal, Émile, 160
Leighton, Douglas, 29
Lekwammen, 78
Lethbridge (AB), 9, 49, 82, 117, 124, 160
Letter Leaflet, 74-75. *See also* Women's Auxiliary (Anglican Church)
Lewis, Oscar, 42
Lucas, Samuel, 83, 105-6, 147

Lutz, John, 78, 145
Lux, Maureen, 7, 30-31, 55, 84-85, 96, 108, 110, 133, 155, 158; *Medicine That Walks*, 30

MacDonald, Sir John A., 84-85
Maclean, Rev. John, 37-39, 58, 63-64, 71, 75, 79; "Blackfoot Medical Priesthood," 38
Maclean, Sarah Anne, 79
Macleod, James, 29
Macleod, Norman Thomas, 29-30
Malainey, Mary, 19
manly-hearted women, 23
Marett, R.R., 13
maternal mortality, 58, 101, 144, 156-57
McBain, Lesley, 101
McClintock, Anne, 9
McClintock, Walter, 37-42, 45; *Old North Trail*, 39, 41
McDougall, Annie, 60, 63
McDougall, Eliza Boyd, 60, 63, 71, 79
McDougall, Rev. John, 60, 63, 70-71, 80
McDougall Residential School, 71, 80, 95, 104, 135
McDowell, Linda, 10
McGill, Dr. Harold, 130, 142
McLaren, Angus, 165
McPherson, Kathryn, 56, 101, 114
measles, 30, 132, 137
medicine bundles, 21, 24, 36, 39, 40, 43
Medicine Hat (AB), 9, 49, 82, 143,
Medicine Hat General Hospital, 82, 97
medicine lodge, 21
medicine men, 35, 38-40, 116, 152, 169
Medicine That Walks (Lux), 30
medicine women, 42, 44, 55, 58, 125-26, 152, 160, 162-64, 166, 168-69
Megarry, Jane, 8, 103, 115-17
Melfort (SK), 56
Methodist National Training School, 108
Methodist Women's Missionary Society, 71
midwifery, 6, 8, 15, 37, 43-45, 48, 50-51, 54-60, 63-64, 68, 87, 143, 152-62, 167. *See also* childbirth; pregnancy
Milloy, John, 104

Index

Misericordia Hospital, 97
Missionary Oblates of Mary Immaculate, 71
Missionary Outlook, 74, 109
missionary work, 6-10, 13-15, 32-33, 36, 47, 51, 58, 60, 63-70, 73-76, 79-83, 85-87, 89-95, 97-105, 112, 118-19, 121-22, 129, 131, 134, 144, 149, 151-52, 155, 160-61, 169, 171-72, 174-75
Missouri River, 18, 25
Mitchinson, Wendy, 157-58
mobile travelling clinics, 143-44. *See also* travelling nurses *under* nursing
Montreal (QC), 31, 57, 98
Moosomin District, 51
Morley Hospital, 108-9
Morley Reserve, 130-31, 134-35, 146
Morley Residential School, 122, 148
Motoki Society (Old Women's Society), 20
Mott, Ella, 58
Mountain Horse, Mike, 126; *My People the Bloods,* 126
Municipal Hospitalization Plan, 57, 143
Murray, Dr. Thomas, 74, 129
My People the Bloods (Mountain Horse), 126

Nakoda (Stoney), 6, 10, 15, 17-19, 21-22, 25-28, 30, 42, 60, 63, 71, 79, 95, 104, 108-9, 119, 126, 134-35, 146-49, 168, 170
Natal (South Africa), 50, 114
National Women's Auxiliary, 73
Navajo, 113
necromancy, 38-39
Nevitt, Richard, 84
New Westminster (BC), 149
Nez Perce, 24
Nicolet, 14, 112, 137, 139, 141
nicotine poisoning, 137
North Saskatchewan River, 18
North West Mounted Police (NWMP), 28, 32, 47, 55, 63, 65, 67, 82, 84-85
North-West Territories, 51, 73
Norway House (MB), 128

nursing: graduate nurses, 4, 74, 81-82, 87, 89, 91, 94, 98, 105-6, 108-9, 114, 119, 130, 132, 134-35, 138-39, 141, 154, 158, 160, 174; public health nurses, 7, 32, 100, 106, 112, 113-14, 116, 128-29, 132-34, 138, 143-44, 148-49, 152, 158, 172-73; travelling nurses, 143, 147, 149, 151, 173. *See also* mobile travelling clinics
nutrition, 135-36, 138, 144

O'Neil, John, 155
Ojibwa, 40
okan (Sun Dance), 20-21, 64
Old North Trail (McClintock), 39, 41
Old Sun Residential School, 110
Oldman River, 27
opthalmia, 75

Palliser Expedition, 48
Paul, Pauline, 82
Peacock, Sandra Leslie, 41-42
Peigan. *See* Piikani (Peigan) *under* Blackfoot Nation
Peigan Reserve, 32, 71, 73, 75, 80, 85, 90, 93-95, 98, 117, 126, 129-33, 147
Peigan Residential School, 80
Perry, Adele, 79
Peterson, Lester, 53
petroleum, 49
Pheasant Forks, 58
Piikani (Peigan). *See under* Blackfoot Nation
Pincher Creek (AB), 59
Pincher Creek United Church, 63
Porcupine Hills, 27
Port Simpson, 108
potlatch, 64
pregnancy, 45, 47, 137, 147, 149, 152, 154, 156, 160, 166. *See also* childbirth; midwifery
Prince Albert (SK), 84
Pringle, Robert, 146-47
prostitution, 65
Provincial Board of Health (Ontario), 96

Qu'Appelle District, 58

Index

Rahal-Ruffing, Mary Ann, 113-14
Raymond (AB), 124
Red Crow, Agnes, 162
Reed, Hayter, 79, 85-86
Reifel, Nancy, 114, 116
religious organizations: Anglican, 14, 32, 73-75, 80-81, 89-94, 97-98, 100, 110, 112, 129, 131, 134-35, 141; Catholic, 6, 14, 32, 52, 71, 74, 85, 89, 91-92, 94, 98-100, 111-12, 118, 141, 159-60, 174; Methodist, 32, 58, 60, 69-71, 74, 79, 89, 93, 95, 104, 108, 122, 135; Protestant, 6, 69-70, 93, 97-99, 118, 142, 160, 174. *See also* missionary work
Report of the British Association for the Advancement of Science, 169
residential schools, 32, 71-74, 94, 96-97, 104-8, 132, 153, 158, 171, 173-74
rheumatism, 35, 75, 137
Richardson, Jane, 125, 159, 161
Richardson, Sharon, 156
Rivers, Dr. J.H., 124
Rocanvalle District, 57
Rocky Mountain House, 24
Royal Jubilee Hospital, 98
Rumney, Alice, 104
Rundle, Robert T., 58, 69
Rupert's Land, 28
Rutherdale, Maya, 9, 51, 102
Rutherford, Bella, 81

Sacred Heart Residential School, 71
Sarcee. *See* Tsuu T'ina (Sarcee)
Sarcee Reserve, 27, 30, 32, 60, 73, 81, 93-95, 105, 112, 129, 132-34, 136-38, 146-48
Sarcee Residential School, 73-74, 94, 113, 129, 134, 137
Saskatchewan Archives Board, 56-57
Sayese, Harriet, 55-56
scarlet fever, 132-33
Schaeffer, Claude, 164-66
Schultz, James Willard, 37, 41
scientific motherhood, 105, 145, 152
Scott, Duncan Campbell, 86, 96, 123, 126, 128, 132, 135, 144, 146-47

Scott-Brown, Joan, 22, 42, 126, 168
Scott's Creek, 27
scrofula, 80, 84, 91, 124, 126, 133-34
Sechelt Nation, 53
Second World War, 22, 31, 130, 157, 167, 173
Shade, Allen, 162
Sheriff, Barbara, 19
Shewell, Hugh, 30; *Enough to Keep Them Alive,* 30
Shoshone, 24
Sifton, Clifford, 96
Siksika (Blackfoot). *See under* Blackfoot Nation
Silverman, Eliane, 60
Similkameen Valley, 53
Sioux-Nakoda Nation, 18
Sisters of Charity, 82, 71, 91, 118, 137, 141, 159, 172. *See also* Grey Nuns
Smallboy, Ellen, 56, 58
smallpox, 30, 84, 109, 132
Smith, Andrea, 64, 171
Smith, Rose Marie, 58-59
Smith, Sherry, 37
Smith, Susan, 50
Social Organization and Ritualistic Ceremonies of the Blackfoot Indian (Wissler), 44
Society for the Promotion of Christian Knowledge, 94
St. Albert (AB), 82, 111, 160
St. Catharine's (ON), 97
St. Joseph's Industrial School, 71, 109
St. Mary River, 26
St. Paul's Residential School, 74, 115
Standoff (AB), 129
Stefansson, Vilhjalmur, 13
Stillborne, Edith Mary, 58
Stocken, Catherine, 73, 75, 106
Stocken, Rev. H.W. Gibbon, 73-74, 90, 98, 117
Stoler, Ann Laura, 8, 87
Stone, Dr. E.L., 127-28, 137
Stoney. *See* Nakoda (Stoney)
Stoney Reserve, 32, 73, 79, 80, 93, 95, 104, 123, 129, 132, 146-47, 149
Storer, Effie, 52-53, 55

Index

Strong-Boag, Veronica, 56
Sundstrom, Linea, 25
syphilis, 84

Taber (AB), 49
Takes Gun on Top, Jappy, 164
Taylor, Winnifred, 58
Thibault, Jean-Baptiste, 69
Thompson, Kay, 55
Thomson, Gerald, 149
Tims, Rev. J.W., 74, 81, 73, 92, 112-13, 134, 137
Toronto (ON), 57, 155
Toronto Women's Auxiliary, 73, 92, 102, 107
trachoma, 106, 136, 172
transcultural nursing, 113-16
Treaty 7, 3-6, 8, 10, 12-13, 15, 17, 25-30, 45, 48-49, 63, 73, 78-79, 81-84, 89, 93-94, 98, 100-1, 106-9, 116, 118-23, 125-26, 128-29, 133, 136, 139, 143, 148, 152-54, 156, 158, 162-63, 172, 174
Trigger, Bruce, 24
Trivett, Samuel, 74
Tsattine, 18
Tsuu T'ina (Sarcee), 6, 10, 13-15, 17-19, 21-22, 24-28, 30-31, 60, 73, 90, 94, 119, 130, 135, 161, 169-70
tuberculosis, 7, 25, 30-31, 53, 74, 94-97, 106-8, 126, 129, 133-34, 136-38, 172
Turner, Alice, 98, 102, 107
Turner, Isabel, 98, 102, 110
two-spirits, 23
typhoid, 149

United Farm Women of Alberta, 154

United Farmers of Alberta, 143
United Farmers of Manitoba, Women's Branch, 57

Valverde, Mariana, 152
Vancouver (BC), 56, 149
Vancouver General Hospital, 56
Vegerville (AB), 143
Victoria (BC), 98
Victoria Home Hospital, 94
Victoria Jubilee Home, 90

Waldram, James, 100
Wall, Dr. J.J., 135
whiskey trade, 25
White, Mary, 160
White, Pamela, 156
White Elk, Mary, 125
Whitefish Lake, 55
whooping cough, 30, 132
Wilson, Rev. E.F., 169
Windsor, Dr. Evelyn, 140, 159
Winnipeg (MB), 59, 82
Wissler, Clark, 12, 38-39, 43-45, 163; *Social Organization and Ritualistic Ceremonies of the Blackfoot Indian,* 44
Wolseley (SK), 55
Women's Auxiliary (Anglican Church), 74, 98
Women's Missionary Society, 79, 93, 95, 108
Wright, Helen, 148

Yaktonai Dakota, 18
Young, Egerton Ryerson, 64
Young, T. Kue, 100, 127

Printed and bound in Canada by Friesens
Set in Garamond by Artegraphica Design Co. Ltd.
Copy editor and proofreader: Lesley Erickson
Cartographer: Eric Leinberger